Locker Tales

Locker Tales
Coffee Beans To Fitness Dreams
Politics to Pandemics

written by Lew Freimark

with major illustrations
by Andrew Arcangeli

and other illustrations
by Peter Campbell

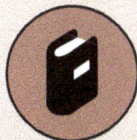

Dance to the Sun Publishers, LLC
ADULT DIVISION

Locker Tales – Coffee Beans To Fitness Dreams - Politics to Pandemics
ISBN: 978-0-9993 110-6-6
Copyright ©2020 by Lewis B. Freimark. All rights reserved.

This novel is a work of historical fiction. Names, descriptions, entities and incidents included in the story are products of the author's imagination. Any resemblance to actual persons, events and entities is entirely coincidental.

The opinions expressed by the author are not necessarily those of
Dance to the Sun Publishers, LLC.

Published by Dance to the Sun Publishers, LLC.
P.O. Box 965, Belle Mead, New Jersey 08502 USA
201-694-9902 | www.soccertales.net

Dance to the Sun Publishers, LLC, is committed to excellence in the publishing field.
As educators and publishers we should help people to understand the issues and history of the day.

Book design: copyright ©2020 Dance to the Sun Publishers, LLC. All rights reserved.
Book cover & interior design and layout: Bill Thauer / CapeWorksWRT.com • capewrt@mac.com
Main illustrations: Andrew Arcangeli, unless otherwise noted
Oher illustrations: Peter Campbell, as noted
Photographs provided by: Lewis Freimark, unless otherwise noted
Cover photo collage: Bill Thauer

Published in the United States of America
ISBN: 978-0-9993 110-6-6

1. Health
2. Fitness
3. Gender & Sexuality
5/4/20

DEDICATION

This book is dedicated to my sons, Jon and Joshua who have made fitness a part of their personal lives.

In Jon's case he has played Division I soccer and run marathons.

Josh has had to overcome serious injuries sustained in a car accident several years ago.

Despite these physical handicaps, he strove to study and become a Certified Personal Trainer under the National Academy of Sports Medicine.

He has worked his way back into physical shape through this training.

He is now studying the art of Jiu-Jitsu in an effort to achieve balance in his life. This is his end game and his ritual for fitness.

I commend them both for their many efforts and acomplishments.

Table Of Contents

Chapter 1

Fitness and Modern Times

Your doctor chides you for being what he deems to be obese. With incredulity you immediately respond with, NO, that can't be me! In my mind's eye, I am still a lean, mean fighting machine.

What is a working definition of obesity? More than average fatness, an encumbrance of flesh. In German it is called: Fettleibigkeit (sounds nasty), in French it is called: obésité (better, used with soft accents), in Spanish it is called sobrepeso (sounds like a pharmaceutical or serious money).[1]

Your mind wanders back to that snapshot of you, playing high school and college basketball 50 years ago or arguing with your boxing buddies about the best fights of the 70s and 80s as if you could still challenge for the heavyweight championship. After watching Muhammad Ali all those years my friends and

I joked around about how I could get in the ring with either Klitschko brother and hold my own. Since Vitali has been elected twice as mayor of Kiev and now heads up the parliamentary party, Ukrainian Democratic Alliance for Reform (UDAR),[2] maybe he should have gotten in the Ukrainian political ring, as the 'Ironfist' and straightened out the Trump mess over the U.S. aid to Ukraine. So we wouldn't have to sell the house with these impeachment proceedings, Vitali!!

So now back on topic you ask yourself the question of how did you put on this weight and now, more importantly, what can you do to shed it?

So one way is to hit the gym or another is to dive into the pool.

"Hey, Bro are you using that machine or what?" The two musclebound trainers were interrogating me while staring and glaring in an ominous manner. "Hey," I answered trying to be as witty as possible, "I didn't know I was so popular." In today's world, the habit of fitness is perceived as the means to overcome our own End Game, which unfortunately is obesity and, as today's medical community points out to us on many TV commercials our own mortality. Let's look at the history and timeline of fitness, mix in some cultural aspects and politicking so that we can better comprehend our struggle with the issues and how we got to where we are today. Let us look at how achieving fitness can be an end game unto itself without the peception of mortality.

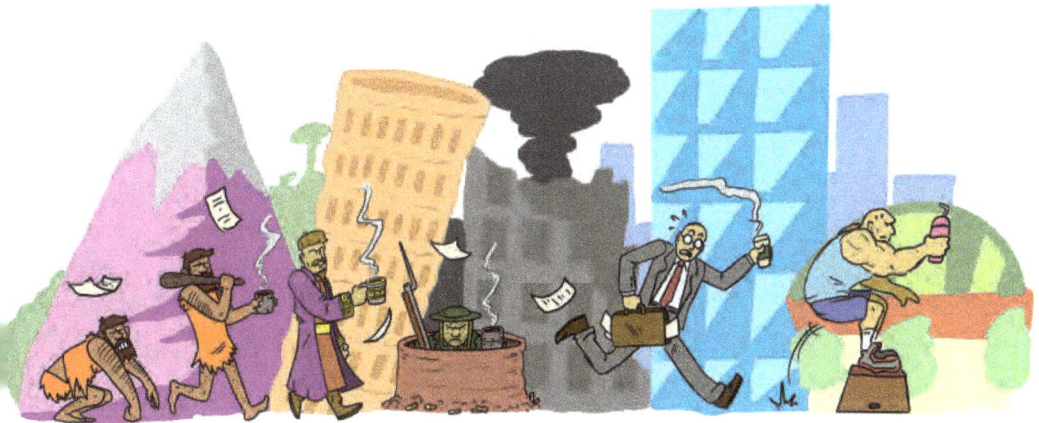

Time Line of Fitness
Throughout Civilization –
Brontosaurus, Bayonet and Board Room

Chapter 2

Caveman and Medieval Fitness

The strength and mobility of early man was not developed through structured programs, methods, or schedules [on fitness machines], but rather was forged by the daily, instinctive, necessity-driven practice of highly practical and adaptable movement skills. Ancient man sought new territories to live in as climate changed. Today, the few hunter-gatherer tribes which still exist around the world would have no idea what "primal fitness" or "caveman workouts" are, as this kind of "exercise" remained deeply ingrained in their everyday lives.[3]

An extreme example of their lack of concern for structured fitness programs was the so-called "Iceman" Ötzi (German) pronunciation: [œtsi], also called the Iceman or the Similaun Man, discovered in the Tyrolean Mountains bordering Austria and Italy in 1991.

This man, dating back 5,000 years, continued to hunt for his family's food, despite having been sick on numerous occasions in his last 6 months of life.

One of his fingernails (of the two found) shows three Beau's lines indicating he was sick three times in the six months before his demise. The last incident, two months before he died, lasted about two weeks. In 2001, X-rays and a CT scan revealed that Ötzi had an arrowhead lodged in his left shoulder. Can you imagine that this guy struggled on for 6 months before he finally fell? The Iceman did not complain as he sought to survive. Further research found that the arrow's shaft had been removed. It is quite possible that he pulled it out himself before death. A close examination of the body found bruises and cuts to the hands, wrists and chest and cerebral trauma indicative of a blow to the head.[4] One can only speculate how modern man would deal with these same survival issues.

Interesting enough with the melting polar ice cap at the North Pole and the Northwest Passage now accessible for oil and gas exploration by competing countries, we are

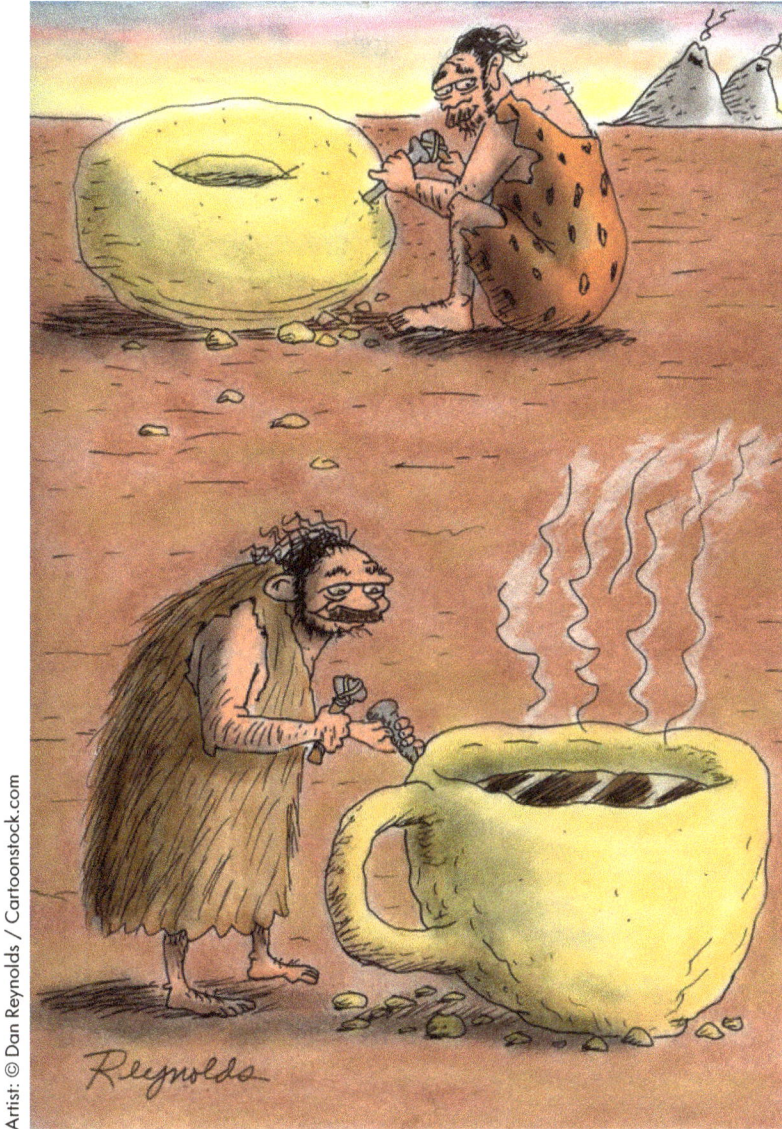

Chiseling cavemen who augur the future.

training our soldiers with the help of the Inuit tribesmen of the north in survival techniques such as navigating and building ice caves, hunting and fishing.[5,6]

When you look at the cross-fitness devotees today such as Katrin Davidsdottir she will tell you that most of these athletes endure the pain of training to get to some beautiful flow state. For these athletes the pain is the reward. These women from Iceland are bridging the gap between their medieval heritage of 930 A.D., when they fled Norway to live a life of endurance on volcanic rock while facing starvation, to today's quest for fitness perfection that they are seeking.[7,8] I would say for most of us this is truly an example of an end game. She truly enjoys her fitness today.

Medieval man fought equally for purposes of religion and the conquest of new lands. Under feudalism, the dominant social system in medieval Europe, only nobles and mercenaries underwent physical training for military service. Similarly to ancient times of Greece and Rome, their training centered on natural movements and martial skill. The rest of the population were mostly peasants obliged to live on their lord's land and work extremely hard in fields using rudimentary tools. Their "exercise" came through hard labor.

Lasting until 1400 A.D., the Middle Ages were a chaotic period with a succession of kingdoms and empires, hordes of barbarian invasions, and devastating plagues. The teachings of Christianity spread the belief that the primary concern of one's lifetime was preparing for the afterlife. In this time the body was seen as primarily sinful and unimportant – it was a man's soul that was his true essence. Education was overwhelmingly connected to the Church, and focused on cultivating the mind rather than training the body.[9]

Chapter 3

Fitness and the Renaissance

Men of the Renaissance and Enlightenment learned and taught the scientific method and rational analysis of the world through empirical study and observation. The Renaissance Era (from around 1400 to 1600) prompted a much greater and open interest in the body, anatomy, biology, health, and physical education.

In 1420, Vittorino da Feltre, an Italian humanist and one of the first modern educators, opened a very popular school where, beyond the humanist subjects, a special emphasis was placed on physical education.[10]

Modern man uses the mind and the development of technology to further his existence. He follows routines to combat the aging process. Man has always been a creature of habit but now it is felt that we can slow the aging process through fitness, nutrition and medical science. Despite all this, the world has measurable limits as we struggle against our own Fettleibigkeit. Now man can empirically comprehend these limitations and use science to strive to overcome the inevitable End Game.

Chapter 4

The Coffee Bean Meets the Age of Enlightenment

The coffee bean was a discovery that helped to expand those measurable limits of human existence. It serviced the leisure class in Europe during the Age of Enlightenment. As the middle class came into existence in Europe in the 16th and 17th centuries people grew fond of spices and coffee beans for their tea and coffee. Merchants became pre-occupied with business and trade for their products and these products spread across the ocean with the landed gentry. The spread of coffee to the rest of the world took place in the seventeenth century. To maintain their monopoly on its control, coffee merchants in Mocha prohibited the distribution of live seeds or seedlings of the coffee plant. This technique worked to restrict coffee production to Yemen (and to restrict coffee distribution to

Mocha) until late in the seventeenth century. This is not to say, however, that other people were unaware of coffee's existence. The British East India company was founded in 1600 to facilitate trade in luxury goods from Asia, particularly spices. By 1620 the British were trading in coffee.[11]

Earlier eras were too busy exploring, fighting wars or maintaining survival mode to worry about growing old and issues of obesity and mortality. Mortality rates were high even if you outpaced childhood diseases. No one had the leisure time to really ponder death or to strategize fitness programs to prevent it. Death was an inevitable fact of life.

The coffee bean then became a fixture of modern times, as man realized he was mortal but sought to prolong his existence through coffee's stimulus and to become even more productive to society.

Chapter 5

The Coffee Bean Meets Yankee Doodle

The coffee bean and its grinding pot were seen as necessities of war and territorial expansion until they reached modern day's corporate America. The battles of the American Revolution started the coffee bean on its historical journey. The *Boston Globe*, on September 11, 2014, advised us that George Washington was a coffee drinker – and an importer. According to his papers and ledger sheets, he imported 200 pounds of coffee in 1770. "I will thank you also for sending me, if an opportunity should offer soon by Water, one hundred weight, or even a Barrel of good Coffee," he wrote in 1784 to a Philadelphia merchant who helped him import goods. In November 1799, just weeks before he died, he asked for 150 beans from the Red Sea port of Mocha, which at the time was considered the best [quality bean].[12]

One can only imagine that when Colonel Henry Knox brought the 59 cannon of Fort Ticonderoga down to Boston during January of 1776, through Lake George and the blinding and windswept winter snows of upstate New York it was likely that provisions of coffee beans helped to sustain the soldiers. Those soldiers conveyed the ox-drawn sled and 60 tons of cannon and other armaments across some 300 miles (480 km) of ice-covered rivers and snow-draped Berkshire mountains to the Boston siege camps. The region was lightly populated and Knox had to overcome difficulties hiring personnel and draft animals. On several occasions cannon crashed through the ice on river crossings, but the detail's men were always able to recover them. In the end, what Knox had expected to take just two weeks actually took more than six, and he was finally able to report the arrival of the weapons train to Washington, in Boston and Dorchester Heights, on January 27, 1776. This event was called by historian Victor Brooks "one of the most stupendous feats of logistics"[13] of the entire war. It is said he [Knox] took on what some deemed to be a 'suicide mission.'

Henry Knox is the Founding Father they don't teach you about in elementary school. Because he was way too much of a 'bad ass.' He wasn't much for signing documents or paying visits to France in frilly shirt cuffs. He was more about firing giant cannon right into the bad guys' faces. Colonel Knox was an artillery guy, you see... the man who made things go BOOM! And when he ran out of guns and cannon, he set up the country's first arsenal in Massachusetts to produce even more. Away from the fighting, he was a stalwart confidante for General Washington and a disciplined organizer of men and provisions.[14]

Knox's effort is commemorated by a series of plaques marking the Henry Knox Trail in New York and Massachusetts.[15]

Lucy and Henry Knox had actually first met in 1774 at Boston coffee shops as their love letters explain. Coffee was a part of their life and very well may have accompanied the colonel and his soldiers on the march to and from Fort Ticonderoga.[16] There is a company today named "The Knox Trail Coffee Company" which operates in the town of Otis, Massachusetts. They are a family run, veteran owned small business, exceedingly passionate about their community and about ALL

THINGS COFFEE! "Our mission they say is to share this passion with all of you. COFFEE LOVERS UNITE!"[17]

Coffee was frequently used by the colonists in America to avoid paying tax on tea shipped from England. Also, note that coffee and coffee houses were locations used for strategizing in the American revolutionary era. As far as coffee house vs. tavern, a coffee house was especially known as a place to conduct business without the distraction of alcohol. That said, an owner still had to serve some alcohol to stay in business. But there were special rooms that were solely designated "coffee only". Socially, I would say the coffee house catered more to the decision makers and were also known to double as a courthouse.

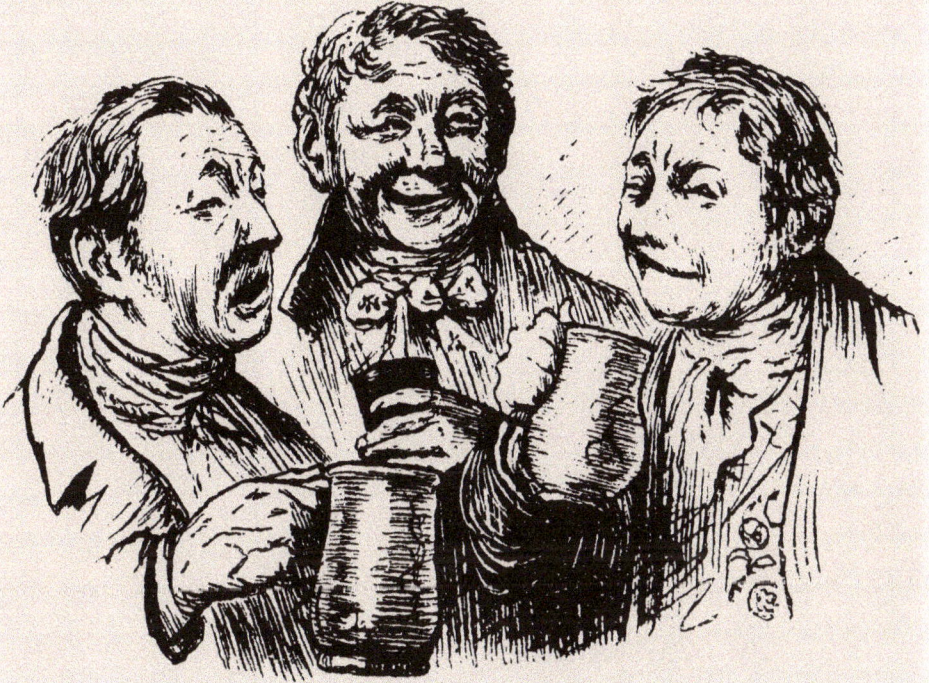

Antique engraving vectorized by: Eric Fritz

COLONIALS ENJOYED THEIR BEVERAGES

These chaps are two and a half sheets to the wind, on their way to a trifecta. Three colonial revolutionaries planning freedom from the British Empire? Three old friends drinking to what was and what will be? Perhaps a spat about the local state of business affairs? The choice is ale or coffee.

Chapter 6

The Coffee Bean Helps Unify the Country

The Civil War was fought on the grim and dusty battlefields of Antietam, Gettysburg and Sharpsburg in Virginia and Maryland. Soldiers wearing heavy wool uniforms, escorted their mule trains and railroad transports dragging heavy cannon into positions in the summers of 1862 and 1863. These tactics would never have proved conclusive without sound field strategies devised by opposing Generals Grant, McClellan, Lee and their officers over tins of coffee.

This author's research has disclosed that General George Crook, who later gained fame during the Civil War, was stationed at Fort Jones. It is said that officers Ulysses S. Grant and Phillip Sheridan were also assigned duty at Fort Jones but never arrived.[18] One can only speculate as to whether Sheridan and Grant

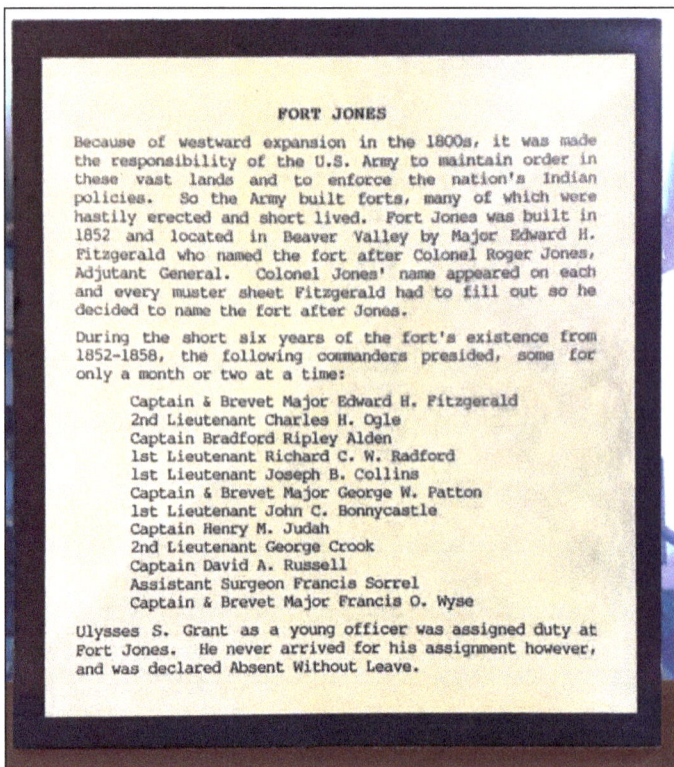

FORT JONES

Because of westward expansion in the 1800s, it was made the responsibility of the U.S. Army to maintain order in these vast lands and to enforce the nation's Indian policies. So the Army built forts, many of which were hastily erected and short lived. Fort Jones was built in 1852 and located in Beaver Valley by Major Edward H. Fitzgerald who named the fort after Colonel Roger Jones, Adjutant General. Colonel Jones' name appeared on each and every muster sheet Fitzgerald had to fill out so he decided to name the fort after Jones.

During the short six years of the fort's existence from 1852-1858, the following commanders presided, some for only a month or two at a time:

Captain & Brevet Major Edward H. Fitzgerald
2nd Lieutenant Charles H. Ogle
Captain Bradford Ripley Alden
1st Lieutenant Richard C. W. Radford
1st Lieutenant Joseph B. Collins
Captain & Brevet Major George W. Patton
1st Lieutenant John C. Bonnycastle
Captain Henry M. Judah
2nd Lieutenant George Crook
Captain David A. Russell
Assistant Surgeon Francis Sorrel
Captain & Brevet Major Francis O. Wyse

Ulysses S. Grant as a young officer was assigned duty at Fort Jones. He never arrived for his assignment however, and was declared Absent Without Leave.

Photo of display board taken by the museum curator, Cecelia Reuter, at Fort Jones Museum, Fort Jones, California November 8, 2019.

knew they would be part of a greater end game. We do know that Generals Grant, Sheridan and Sherman would strategize during these military campaigns over their favorite cigars and strong coffee. Grant would abstain from any alcoholic beverage because of his past drinking history and would consume coffee for his frequent bouts of headaches.

In their struggle against mortality at the horrific battle at Antietam it was transformed

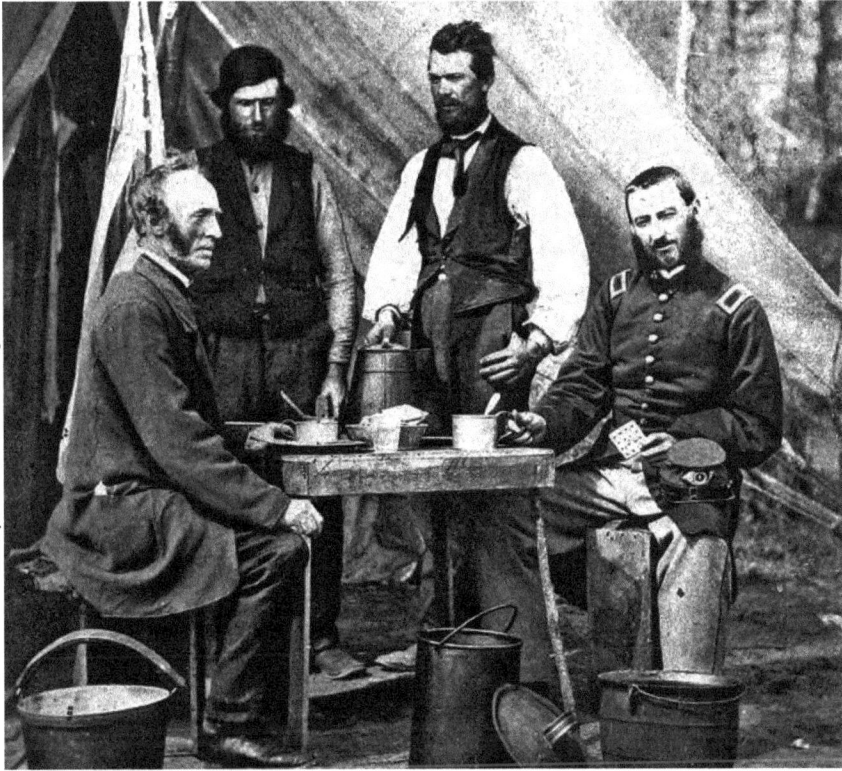

PHOTO: James F. Gibson / May, 1862, Yorktown, Virginia area

Strategizing on a Civil War battlefield with a tin of coffee and rations.
Union soldier, Ebenezer Nelson Gilpin, wrote in his diary in 1865:
"...No one can soldier without coffee."

into the greatest coffee run in American history. The Ohio boys had been fighting since morning, trapped in the raging battle in September, 1862. Suddenly, a 19-year-old William McKinley appeared, under heavy fire, hauling vats of hot coffee. The men held out tin cups, gulped the brew and started firing again. "It was like putting a new regiment in the fight," their officer recalled [they were energized into their fighting fitness with the use of coffee]. Three decades later, McKinley ran for president in part on this singular act of caffeinated heroism. The bean had, again, bequeathed its life-support to the fighting men of America.

At the time, no one found McKinley's act all that strange. For Union soldiers, and the lucky Confederates who could scrounge some, coffee fueled the war. Soldiers drank it before marches, after marches, on patrol, and during combat. In their diaries, "coffee" appears more frequently than the words "rifle," "cannon" or "bullet." Ragged veterans and tired nurses agreed with one diarist: "Nobody can 'soldier' without coffee." Coffee, and its power of energizing the soldiers to keep them fighting, became a staple of combat.

Union troops made their coffee everywhere, and with everything: with water from canteens and puddles, brackish bays and Mississippi mud: water that their horses would not drink. They cooked it over fires of plundered fence rails, or heated mugs in scalding steam-vents on naval gunboats. When times were good, coffee accompanied beefsteaks and oysters; when they were bad it washed down raw salt-pork and maggoty hardtack. Coffee was often the last comfort troops enjoyed before entering battle, and the first sign of safety for those who survived their own mortality. Coffee was the elixir of fitness for both sides during modern warfare.

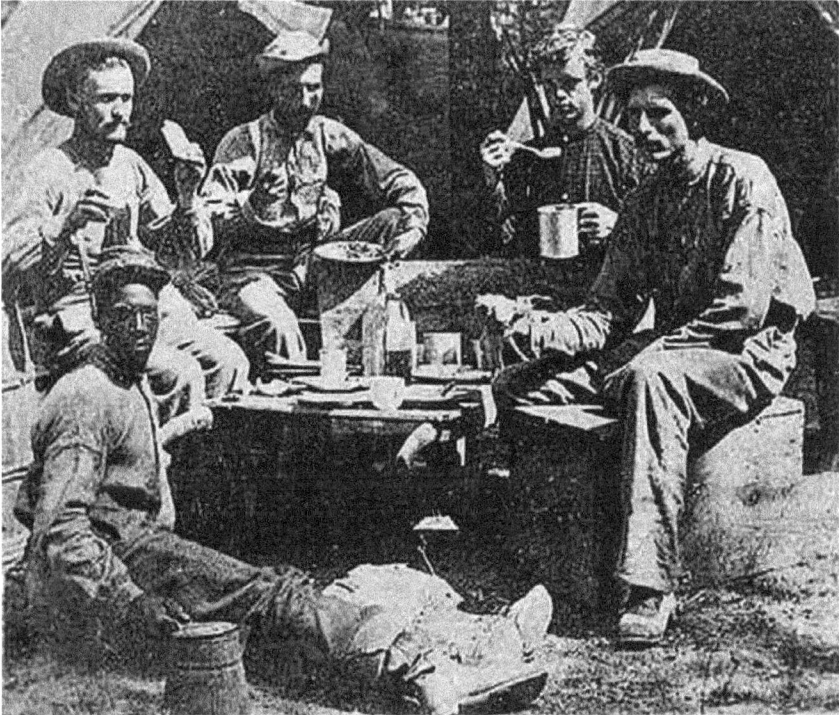

PHOTO: library of Congress

TOOTHDULLERS AND SKILLYGALEE.
MEALTIME IN THE CIVIL WAR.
Hardtack could be eaten plain, though most men preferred to toast them over a fire, crumble them into soups, or fry them with their pork and bacon fat in a dish called skillygalee. Coffee was a most important staple, and some soldiers considered it (and sugar) more important than anything else.

The Union Army encouraged this love, issuing soldiers roughly 36 pounds of coffee each year. Men ground the beans themselves (some carbines even had built-in grinders) and brewed it in little pots called muckets. They spent much of their downtime discussing the quality of that morning's brew. Reading their diaries, one can sense the delight (and addiction) as troops gushed about a "delicious cup of black," or fumed about "wishy-washy coffee." Escaped slaves who joined Union Army camps could always find work as cooks if they were good at "settling" the coffee – getting the grounds to sink to the bottom of the unfiltered muckets.The coffee was seen as extending the soldier's life allowing the troops to continue their day-to-day existence.

For much of the war, the massive Union Army of the Potomac made up the second-largest population center in the Confederacy, and each morning this sprawling city became a coffee factory. First, as another diarist noted, "little campfires, rapidly increasing to hundreds in number, would shoot up along the hills and plains." Then the encampment buzzed with the sound of thousands of grinders simultaneouly crushing beans. Soon tens of thousands of muckets gurgled with fresh brew.

Confederates were not so lucky. The Union blockade kept most coffee out of seceded territory. One British observer noted that the loss of coffee "afflicts the Confederates even more than the loss of spirits," while an Alabama nurse joked that the fierce craving for caffeine would, somehow, be the Union's "means of subjugating us." When coffee was available, captured or smuggled or traded with Union troops during casual cease-fires, Confederates wrote rhapsodically about their first sip. The absence of the bean was seen as a destroyer of life itself for the struggling Confederate army.

Sometimes the problem spilled over to the Union invaders. When Gen. William T. Sherman's Union troops decided to live off plunder

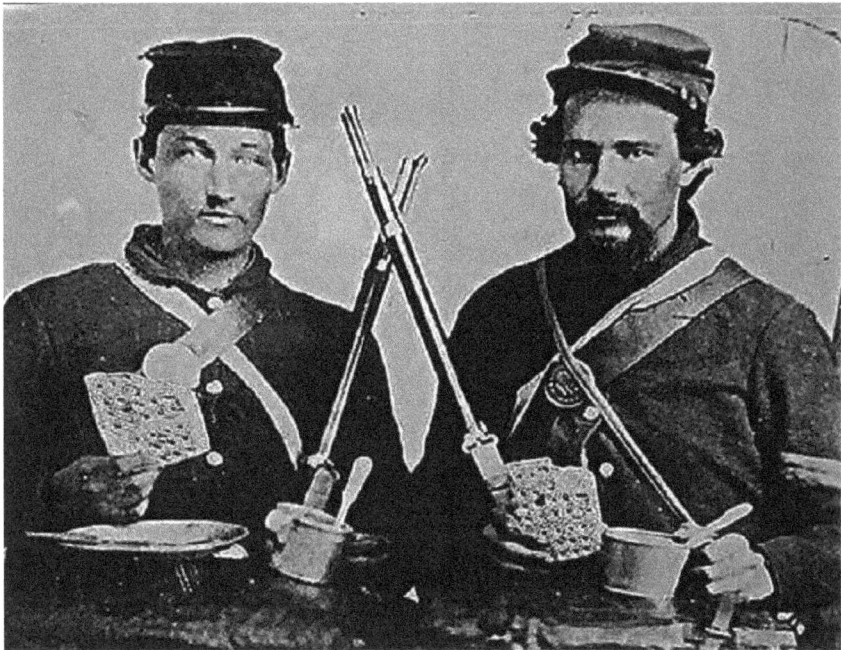

PHOTO: Courtesy of the James C. Fresca Collection

Two Ohio Union soldiers enjoying their ration of hardtack.

and forage as they cut their way through Georgia and South Carolina, soldiers complained that while food was plentiful, there were no beans to be found. "Coffee is only got from Uncle Sam," an Ohio officer grumbled, and his men "could scarce get along without it."

Confederate soldiers and civilians would not fight without some form of coffee. It was seen as a necessity to continue their energy and fighting spirit. So both sides saw coffee as a necessity of war in keeping the soldiers' combat readiness. Many cooked up coffee substitutes, roasting corn or rye or chopped beets, grinding them finely and brewing up something warm and brown. It contained no caffeine, but desperate soldiers claimed to love it. Gen. George Pickett, famous for that failed charge at Gettysburg, thanked his wife for the delicious "coffee" she had sent, gushing: "No Mocha or Java ever tasted half so good as this rye-sweet-potato blend!"

Did the fact that Union troops were near jittery from coffee, while rebels survived on impotent brown water, have an impact on the outcome of the conflict? Union soldiers certainly thought so. Though they rarely used the word "caffeine" in their letters and diaries they raved about that "wonderful stimulant in a cup of coffee," considering it a "nerve tonic." One depressed soldier wrote home that he was surprised that he was still living, and reasoned: "what keeps me alive must be the coffee."[19] This is another testament to the energy qualities of the elixir.

Others went further, considering coffee a weapon of war. Gen. Benjamin Butler ordered his men to carry coffee in their canteens, and planned attacks based on when his men would be most caffeinated. He assured another general, before a fight in October 1864, that "if your men get their coffee early in the morning you can hold."

Coffee did not win the war – Union material resources and manpower played a much, much bigger role than the quality of its Java – but it might say something about the victors. From one perspective, coffee was emblematic of the upcoming and modern day corporate-industrial way of life. The new Northern society evinced fast-paced wage labor, a hurried, business-minded, industrializing nation of strivers. For years, Northern bosses had urged their workers to switch from liquor to coffee, dreaming of sober, caffeinated, untiring employees. Southerners drank coffee too – in New Orleans especially – but the way Union soldiers gulped the stuff at every meal pointed ahead toward the world the war had made, a civilization that lived on in modern times in every office breakroom until the fitness room and health club replaced it. [Now the annual 5K run, the treadmill, the step climber and the rowing machine are pivotal to man's current quest for fitness and immortality.]

But more than that, coffee was simply delicious, soothing – "the soldier's chiefest bodily consolation" – for men and women pushed themselves through its use beyond their limits. Soldiers often brewed coffee at the end of long marches, deep in the night while other men assembled tents. These grunts were too tired for caffeine to make a difference; they just wanted to share a warm cup – of Brazilian beans or scorched rye – before passing out.

This explains their fierce love for the bean and how it energized them for the battles they were facing. When one captured Union soldier was finally freed from a prison camp, he meditated on his experiences. Over his first cup of coffee in more than a year, he wondered if he could ever forgive "those Confederate thieves for robbing me of so many precious doses." Getting worked up, he fumed, "Just think of it, in three hundred days there was lost to me, forever, so many hundred pots of good old Government Java."

So when William McKinley braved enemy ire to bring his comrades a warm cup – an act memorialized in a stone monument at Antietam today – he knew what it meant to them.[20]

Chapter 7

The Coffee Bean Tames The Old West

Coffee was also a mainstay of the Old West as our country sought its Manifest Destiny and no cowpoke worth his salt could do without a cup of Arbuckles.'®

Cowboy's First Coffee

When a cowboy had his Arbuckles'® in hand, he was enjoying a cup of coffee.

The Arbuckle Brothers of Pittsburgh made a mighty fine pre-roasted bean that was so popular in the Old West that Arbuckles'® eventually became interchangeable with the actual word coffee, as in "Don't talk to me in the morning until I have my Arbuckles'®" The 'recipe' for coffee was generally a handful of coffee in a cup of water.

Up until the close of the Civil war, coffee

was sold green. It had to be roasted on a wood stove or in a skillet over a campfire before it could be ground and brewed. A single burned bean could ruin the lot.

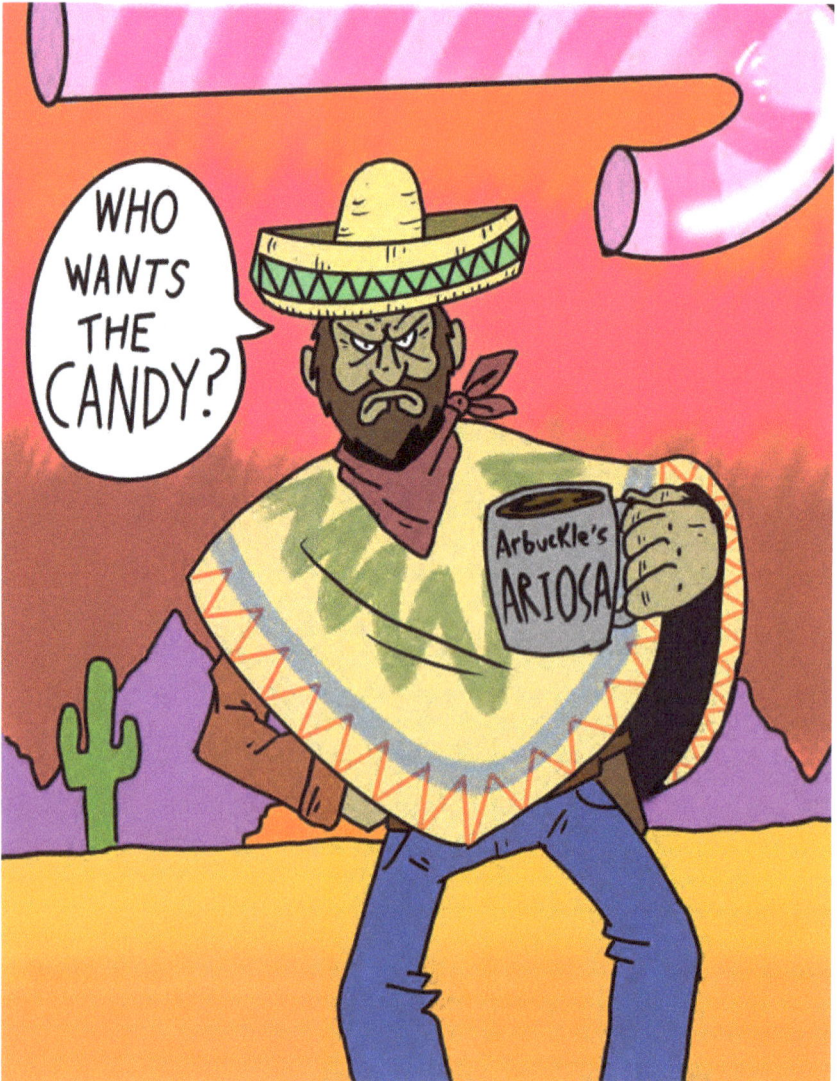

Newsflash! Even Mr. Clint Eastwood, the gruffest, tuffest cowboy wants the candy, a democrat for president, like Mike Bloomberg and he offers props to the *#MeToo Movement*.![21]

In 1865, John Arbuckle and his brother Charles, partners in a Pittsburgh grocery business, changed all this by patenting a process for roasting and coating coffee beans with an egg and sugar glaze to seal in the flavor and aroma. The coffee was marketed under the name Arbuckles.'®

Ariosa® coffee, in airtight packages, was an instant hit with the chuck wagon cooks in the west who were faced with the task of keeping cowboys well fed and supplied with plenty of hot coffee out on the cold range.

Arbuckles'® Ariosa® Coffee packages bore a yellow label with the name Arbuckles' in large red letters across the front, beneath which flew a Flying Angel trademark over the words Ariosa® Coffee in black letters.

It was shipped all over the country in sturdy wooden crates, one hundred packages to a crate. Arbuckles'® Ariosa® coffee became so dominant, particularly in the west, that many cowboys were not even aware there was any other kind.

The Arbuckle Brothers knew they had a good thing going. They printed signature coupons on the bags of coffee redeemable for all manner of items including handkerchiefs, razors, scissors and wedding rings, everything a cowpoke or pioneer might come to need.

To further entice the purchaser, each package of Arbuckles'® contained a stick of peppermint candy. Due to the demands on chuck wagon cooks to keep ready supplies of hot Arbuckles'® on hand around the campfire, the peppermint stick became a means by which that steady coffee supply was ground. Upon hearing the cook's call "Who wants the candy?" some of the toughest cowboys on the trail were known to die for the opportunity of manning the coffee grinder in exchange for satisfying a sweet tooth.

The cowboys' favorite, Arbuckles'® Ariosa® Coffee, is available today, complete with the original Flying Angel trademark. The one pound packages of rich beans remain full-bodied and aromatic. There's still even a piece of peppermint inside.[22]

I remember as a kid that A & P grocery stores also used to grind their own coffee beans. It was called Eight O'Clock® Coffee. Eight O'Clock® Coffee was created by the Great Atlantic & Pacific Tea Company in 1859, in the latter company's founding year. Despite selling off the brand in 2003, A&P continued to sell Eight O'Clock® Coffee in its family of stores until the supermarkets closed in late 2015.[23]

And, of course, who can forget Slim Pickens and the *Blazing Saddles* campfire flatulence scene with the cowboys eating beans and bread, and the big old pot of coffee brewing over the fire? A tradition of the Old West memorialized in cinema by Mel Brooks and produced by Warner Brothers in 1974. In 2006, *Blazing Saddles* was deemed "culturally, historically, and aesthically significant" by the Library of Congress and was selected for preservation in the National Film Registry.

Chapter 8

The Coffee Bean and World War

In World War I, the invention of instant coffee became utilized and helped to defeat the Germans after the United States entered the war.

On April 6, 1917, the U.S. declared war on Germany and formally entered World War I. By late June, American infantry troops began arriving in Europe. One thing they couldn't do without? Coffee, which provided them with the energy to continue to just fight on in the trenches of Europe.

"Coffee was as important as beef and bread," a high-ranking Army official concluded after the war. A postwar review of the military's coffee supply concurred, stating that it "restored courage and strength" and "kept up the morale."

"If *War is Hell*, then coffee has offered U.S. soldiers some salvation." In World War I, the

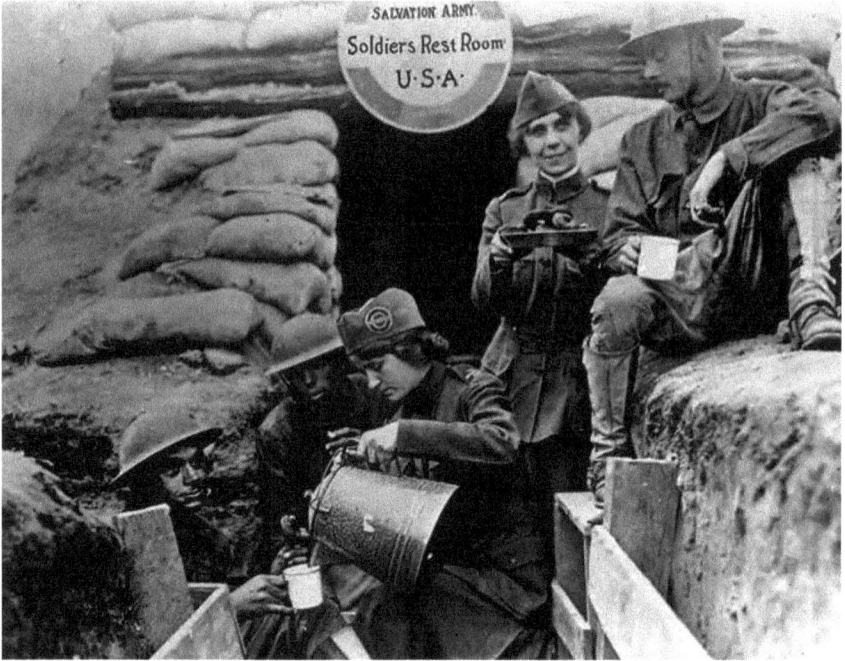

American servicemen enjoying a hot cup of coffee as lassies served doughnuts in the trenches of WWI. A part of Americana that goes well beyond the 'cop on the beat eating donuts.'[24,25] During World War I, instant coffee was a key provision for soldiers on the front.

U.S. War Department took things further, establishing local roasting and grinding plants in France to ensure fresh coffee for the troops. (Even if it was brewed in the worst possible of manners, with the grounds left in the pots for a number of successive meals.) The military also began offering coffee of a different type: instant.

In 1901, a Japanese chemist working in Chicago named Satori Kato developed a successful way to make a soluble coffee powder, or dried coffee extract. At that year's Pan-American Exposition in Buffalo, N.Y., the Kato Coffee Co. served hot samples in the Manufacturers Building, giving the brew its public debut. Two years later Kato received a patent for "coffee concentrate and process of making same."

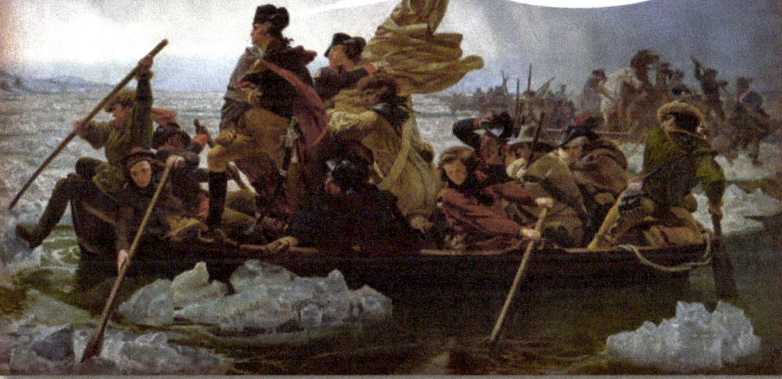

DID YOU KNOW:

George Washington invented instant coffee...

A nice cuppa joe sure would be nice...

Tip of the hat to Emanuel Leuze's *Washington Crossing The Delaware*, 1851.

Yes. But not *that* George Washington. In 1906, a Belgian, also named George Washington, living in Guatemala, was the inventor.

But it was another immigrant in America, an Anglo-Belgian inventor named George Washington, who first successfully mass-produced instant coffee. (Washington's presidential namesake, as previous cited in Chapter 5, was not only a coffee drinker even perhaps an importer.) Established in 1910, the G. Washington Coffee Refining Co., with production facilities in Brooklyn, N.Y., initially sold as "Red E Coffee." Today colleges dining facilities, such as Princeton University, market this coffee as small pouches of "Red Eye® Coffee" through a company named Ellis. Ellis coffees have been family roasted since the company's beginning in 1854 as a shop on Philadelphia's waterfront. Today they package the experience of that shoppe into their single serve coffee cups.[26] The name obviously lends itself to the energy needed for the late night study sessions for college students.

While the name suggested convenience, marketing soon highlighted other benefits of the *perfectly digestible coffee*. "Now you can drink all the COFFEE you wish!" an early 1914 ad in the *New York Times* promised. "No more do you have to risk indigestion when you drink coffee," thanks to a "wonderful process that removes the disturbing acids and oils (always present in ordinary coffee)." Here is an early reference to health aid beyond the elixir's primary purpose of keeping a person awake.

Competing products were hitting the market when demand for soluble coffee skyrocketed with the American entry into the Great War in 1917. The U.S. military snapped up all the instant coffee it could. By October 1918, just before the war's end, Uncle Sam was trying to get 37,000 pounds a day of the powder – far above the entire national daily output of 6,000 pounds, according to Mark Pendergrast's coffee history, *Uncommon Grounds.*[27]

"After trying to put it up in sticks, tablets, capsules and other forms," noted William Ukers in his authoritative *All About Coffee*, "it was determined that the best method was to pack it in envelopes." Each held a quarter ounce.[28] Soluble coffee was notably used on the front lines. Soldiers stirred it into hot water, gulped from tin mugs, and called it "a cup of George," after the company's founder – whose name was apparently familiar to at least some of them.[29]

In a letter from the front that Pendergrast quotes, a soldier wrote: "There is one gentlemen I am going to look up first after I get through helping whip the Kaiser, and that is George Washington, of Brooklyn, the soldiers' friend." The U.S. War Department's E.F. Holbrook, head of the coffee branch of the Subsistence Department, considered instant coffee instrumental in the face of chemical weapons: "The use of mustard gas by the Germans made it one of the most important articles of subsistence used by the army," he explained to the *Tea and Coffee Trade Journal* in 1919. The "extensive use of mustard gas made it impossible to brew coffee by the ordinary methods in the rolling kitchens," he said.

Equally important was coffee's effect on morale in the trenches. It was hot, familiar, and offered a hint of home's comforts. And it had caffeine, which helped energize the troops.

For java addicts like Mexican-American doughboy José de la Luz Sáenz, who served with the 360th Infantry Expeditionary Forces in France and occupied Germany, that jolt also kept at bay "the headaches caused by the lack of coffee in the morning," he wrote in his journal on Sept. 26, 1918, after a sleepless night and gas attack on the Western Front.

Rather than using his 'condiment can' to carry food, he filled one of its compartments with sugar and the other with instant coffee. Managing to get a small alcohol stove to heat water, he prepared cups in the trenches. "The hot coffee with our reliable 'hardtack' biscuits hit the spot, and revived exhausted, hungry, and drowsy soldiers," noted Sáenz, a teacher (and future civil rights activist) from South Texas.

Sometimes Sáenz and his fellow soldiers had to do without heat – or even water – for their coffee. "On occasions when the morning finds us on our feet, I am glad to be able to chew on a spoonful of coffee with a bit of sugar."[30]

EARLY ADVERTISEMNT: New York Tribune / Library of congress – Washington's instant coffee

Bringing coffee home from the battlefield.

After the first world war ended, Washington's company relaunched "prepared coffee" for the household. While Washington's company continued to sell coffee, its Swiss competitor, Nestlé®, managed to develop a better technique for producing instant coffee. In 1938 it launched Nescafé®, which soon dominated the global instant coffee market.

In 1943, just before his death, Washington sold the company. (In 1961, the George Washington coffee brand was discontinued.) By then World War II was raging, and American G.I.s were calling their coffee by a different name: 'Joe.'

GIs enjoyed a cup of coffee during World War II. "The American soldier became so closely identified with his coffee that 'G.I. Joe' gave his name to the brew,"

One legend behind the origins of the new moniker is that it referred to Josephus Daniels, secretary of the Navy from 1913 to 1921 under Woodrow Wilson, who banned alcohol onboard ships, making coffee the strongest drink in the mess. Snopes (debunking site), though, fact-checked that claim and called it false.

Yet 'Joe' very likely does originate in the military. "The American soldier became

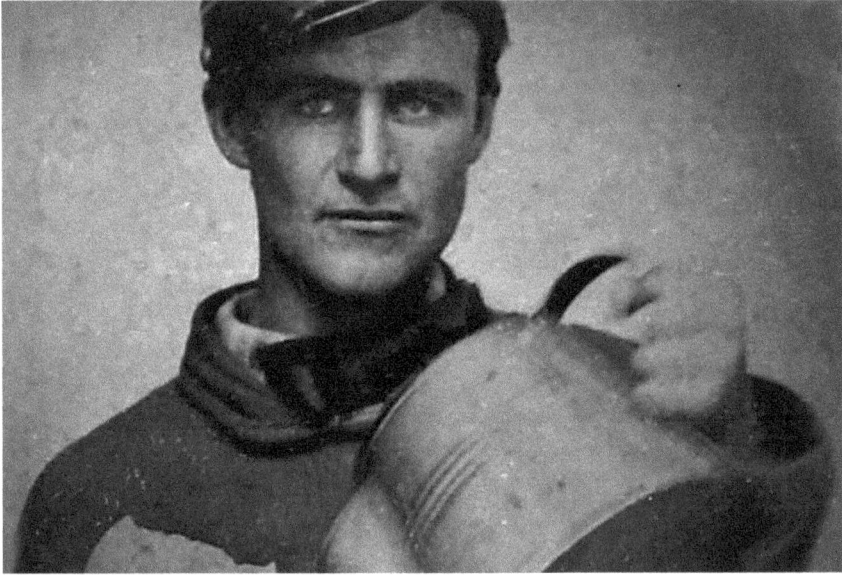

A soldier loves a refreshing cup of coffee
to boost his fitness for battle.

so closely identified with his coffee that G.I. Joe gave his name to the brew," according to Mark Pendergrast.[31]

"Nobody can soldier without coffee," a Union cavalryman had recalled and prophesized for the future while writing in his diary at the end of the Civil War. Many servicemen and women who have fought since then would agree. Even when the coffee was instant and called George.[32]

Chapter 9

Kingpins of the 70s
#Pushback-Brigade
and *#MeToo Movement*

After WW II, the familiar voices of athletes, Jackie Robinson for Chock Full of Nuts® and Joe Dimaggio for Mr. Coffee® highlighted coffee for all folks in America. These coffees were easy to brew for the home and office.

Today's coffee pot constituencies have surrendered their white flag to the fitness routines of the gym and corporate America and are taking no prisoners. No more milling around the office kitchen in the a.m. with a mug of coffee and the light banter of office raconteurs communicating office and personal politics.

In today's busy office setting it is unlikely that someone has taken upon themselves the task of buying the coffee pot, pre-selecting the

the beans, collecting money from users and contributing to the making of that special aroma It is now easier to get to the office with a cup of Peets,® Starbucks® or Lavazza.® It was Howard D. Schultz who picked up on the Italian idea of a coffee bar which would

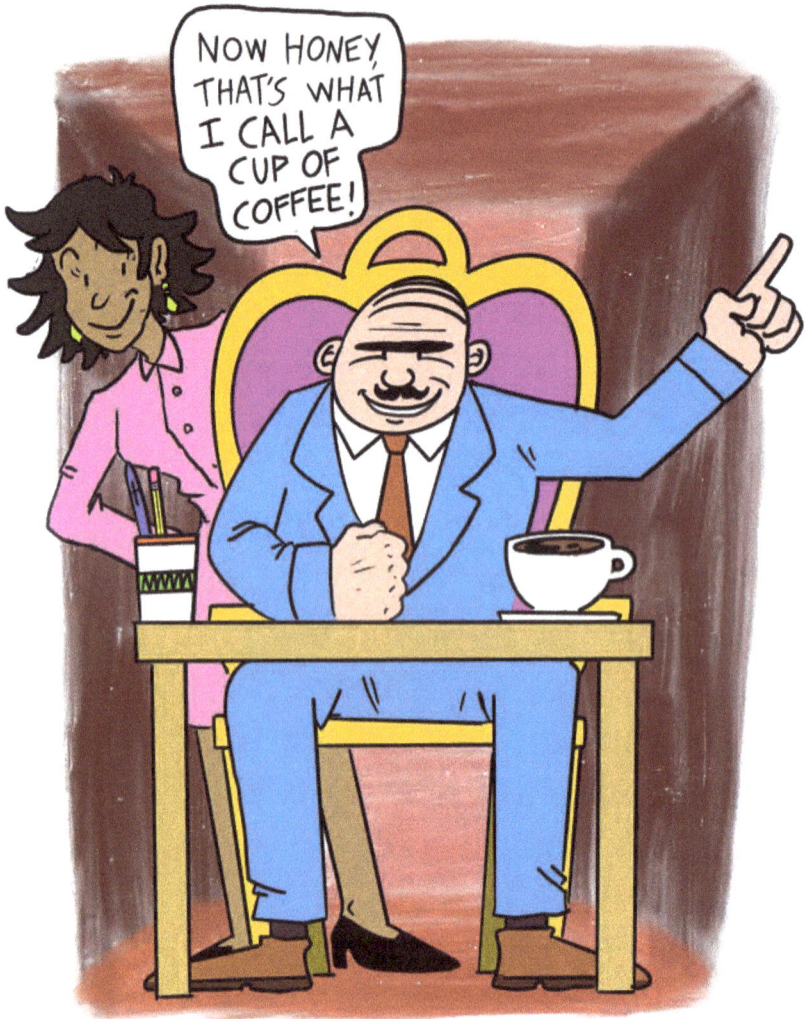

"Coffee for the Kingpin!"

be a meeting place for sipping coffee, and which was located outside of the corporate setting. Now with internet access you can plant yourself at Starbucks® before the office opens. No time to talk about life and the coffee bean like Jerry Seinfeld in Netflix's *Comedians in Cars Getting Coffee.*

In our office my gal Alex kept paying for it out of her own pocket and nobody was contributing to the collection. She finally shut it down and basically told people to get their own damn coffee! You go Alex!

Now I can remember as far back as the 1970s and 80s when I first began working for a large insurance company in Manhattan that the Sunday N.F.L football games were the first order of business on Monday mornings around the pot of coffee. It was part of my comfort zone following a routine of settling into the commute to work. I traveled on the A train from the 178th stop in Washington Heights into lower Manhattan. Many others in the office commuted from Queens and further out in Nassau County.

Sometimes the more aggressive women, like Dana, who did not know anything about football, would try to horn in on the conversation to be competitive with what the office hombres were taking to heart. I, for one, resented them trying to enter our domain. Was it the Giants or Jets who were making up ground on the rest of the league or the battles of the Rangers and Islanders or the Philadelphia Flyers? No one in the brew room kitchen of our office building were fans of the Philly teams. It was like homegrown wars. Throw the Knicks and the 76'ers into the conversation and you had the makings of all-out brawls. Most of the men in our office wore those verbal jousts as scars with pride. Besides Bill Laimbeer and his Bad Boys of the 1989 brawling Detroit Pistons, Michael Jordan and his Chicago Bulls took no back seat in any of those on-court wars.[33]

Yet in its own way, it was comforting to know you could start the work week with those manly conversations. It eased you into the insurance claims that needed to be analyzed throughout the workday. No cell phones or computers were utilized in the offices. We shared an office between Elias a.k.a. Leo, myself, Jeff the Giant, Glen the Delaware Midget, and Freaky Freddy and on Mondays, especially, it was time to go down to Wally Frank's

Ltd. and break open a tin of quality cigars in the office. There were no smoking restrictions in the 70s and the billows of cigar smoke were definitely a way of keeping the women out of our conversations unless it was, of course, Dana. She liked a good cigar. Intractable chauvinism was what I called it, and for guys it was a kind of badge that we wore. This was an age that preceded the *#MeToo* and Fitness Movements. It was the age of Wilt Chamberlain and athletes were the stars until the AIDS crisis struck.

"Far more astonishing in the age of AIDS is the assertion by a player in the NBA's Eastern Conference – not an All-Star, and not yet 30 – who estimates that he has slept with 2,500 different women, and counting. It isn't all boast. There are dozens like him in all the big pro sports. "Let's face it," says Seattle SuperSonics forward Eddie Johnson, "athletes are whores. We're paid to use our bodies. So sex becomes the same thing after the games. We become like dogs sometimes, and we all talk about the same women in every city. Just walk outside the locker room in any arena. The women are all there waiting."[34]

I was one of the kings amidst our court, the secretaries and clerks whom we dated were there and they did not question any of our integrity. It also became the gristmill of our coffee conversations. The ladies were not allowed to participate (except for good old Dana, who we sometimes let in to our clubhouse) and for the time that we lived in that world we most certainly relished our stature.

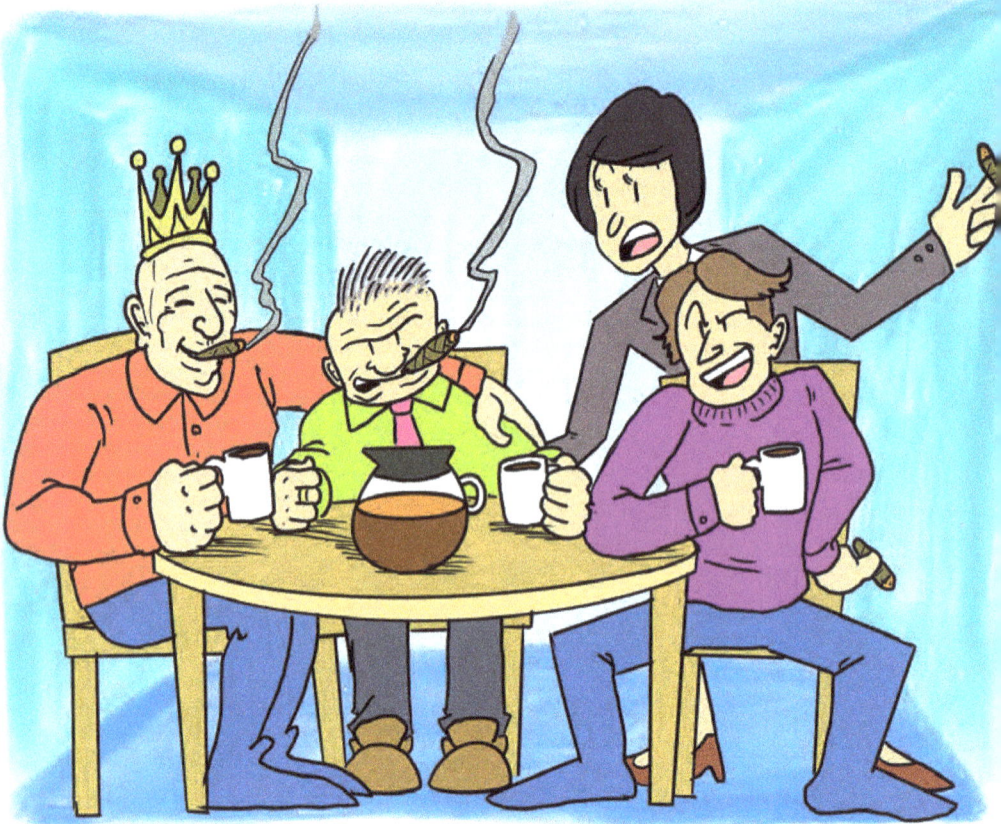

King-Pins of the 70s and lettin' Dana in on the fun.

Nowadays there is pushback by men to the *#MeToo Movement*. Men have to worry about what jokes are made and to understand more about sensitivities. But some of the scenarios have gotten out of control and men today are pushing back. Let me recount some of these episodes I am personally familiar with.

Sam, our very own Oscar, said he had to respond to an employee complaint through his union. The woman said "he was staring at her crotch." Sam told me a butcher's knife had fallen on the floor and he went to retrieve it. Fortunately for him, that case was dismissed by the union board for lack of proof. He could have lost his job. It was a case of she said, he said, as many of them unfortunately are today. However, and in all fairness, 70s and 80s humor is no longer appropriate and men have to be even more sensitive to the *#MeToo Movement*. The *#MeToo Movement* makes a valid point when it comes to exposing inequities in credit scores and lines of credit. AppleCard and Goldman Sachs have been accused of gender inequities in its algorithm. Even Apple co-founder Steve Wozniak complains that his wife's credit line was 10X less than his, even though they have equal assets.[35] I am a true supporter of that movement but I think at times it has gone over the line in terms of sexuality.

I was just recently watching an episode of *24* on Amazon Prime, and Twentieth-Century Fox Television and one of the women analysts, Shari Rothenberg, indicated that a male co-worker had just "brushed by her shoulder" as an innuendo for sexual harassment. This is certainly a teaching moment because *24* was filmed for 18 seasons starting in 2001.

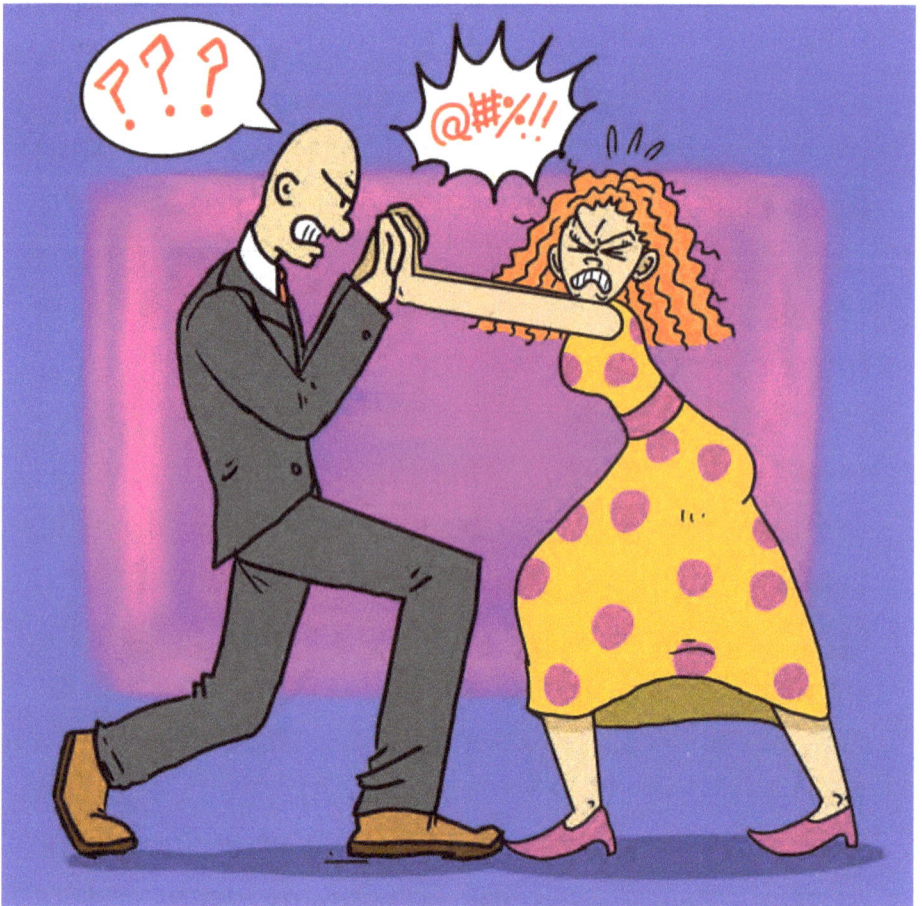

#Push-Back Brigade vs. *#MeToo Movement.*

But the *#MeToo Movement* may also, if it is not careful lose sight of its goals, in its attempt to stabilize gender relations.[36]

The locker room atmosphere itself can be highly charged. An unpleasant incident occurred at my health club. I was falsely accused of stalking a female member. She actually filed a written complaint, and forced me to respond. The problems which ensued were that she talked to the other Wet Team members about it. Fortunately, no one thought her story was credible. It was very embarrassing to hear people discussing this at the club and there were text messages among what we call our Wet Team which caused a chaotic situation.

This was not even remotely a "Matt Lauer or Bill Cosby" situation, and as a side note, and just to show you the accusatory nature of this person, she also accused Veronica of making racially charged comments towards her about not wanting her in the club because she was black. Veronica emphatically denies this accusation and went on record with the club as well. Nothing has been heard back about her charges.

Another guy, Ronnie, at the club tells the tale of how he was jokingly accused by his friends through text messages of having the ability in his home sales to approach women. He was not kidding around in the locker room judging from the look on his face. He confronted the other gym members the next day and taunted back at them, "It's my livelihood, don't kid around about that stuff!"

It is this author's opinion that today these are all examples of too much emphasis placed on gender and racial confrontation.

Now, supporters of the *#MeToo Movement* want to rewrite the lyrics to the classic, Frank Loesser 1944 song, "Baby Its Cold Outside," to avoid any suggestion that a woman may wish to stay at the party with a man that has picked her up. One commentator noted that the new version is basically an attempt to convince us that today a man may choose to kick a woman out of his home though she clearly wants to stay: "When you rewrite the lyrics for the man and leave the woman's basically the same, it really doesn't make any sense. The woman clearly wants to stay. She had a good time, but she's concerned what other people might think. But in this version, the man apparently wants her to go away, but she just won't leave."[37]

We obviously have some high profile celebrity cases like Harvey Weinstein and Jeffrey Epstein where people of substantial power have abused their positions to obtain sexual favors.[38] Harvey Weinstein was convicted on February 24, 2020, in Manhattan, of 3rd degree rape and criminal sexual act, and faces up to 29 years in prison. For the most part we need to pay more attention to people no matter what station in life they fit into and whether the allegations which are hurled at them are substantiated or frivolous.

Surveys taken today show the ambivalence of men towards the *#MeToo Movement* in the *#Push-Back Brigade.*

My guys' generation will tell you that the ladies back in the 70s and 80s were so-o-o beautiful. Stiletto heels, lots of make-up and high skirts. There were mutual affections in the office and everyone understood there was availability for dating. Most of the females in our office did not seem to mind our flirtations at all, in fact they welcomed our advances. There were 3 Spanish olive-skinned beauties assigned to our section and to our hearts' delight. There were Italian and Irish administrative assistants who welcomed our

In a survey conducted by the University of Colorado it was found that: the *#ME TOO MOVEMENT* TRIGGERED GENDER BACKLASH AS MEN TRY TO 'MAINTAIN EXISTING HIERARCHIES OF POWER.' Stefanie Johnson, study co-author and associate professor of organizational leadership and information analytics at University of Colorado Boulder told Newsweek previous studies have shown that sexual harassment has remained relatively constant between 1976 and 2017. She also pointed to data from the Lean In Institute suggesting that *#MeToo* has made men afraid to mentor women to avoid accusations of sexual harassment. "So, we see that *#MeToo* might have changed men's behavior in negative ways (not wanting to mentor women), but what about women? The findings show that women are experiencing less unwanted sexual attention and sexual coercion. Success! But, they reported increased gender harassment, consistent with the mentoring comments." [39,40]

verbal jousting when it came to the weekends. The most magnificent woman of them all for me was the Algerian. Alabaster skin and jet black hair, a body that you would kill for and the French language when she got angry. This was a pretty sultry combination. I will never forget our relationship.

Weekend summer trips and parties to Fire Island as a staff were the cut of the Kingpins' jib. Everyone in the office was subject to being roasted and toasted. The drunker we got the raunchier the stories became. No restrictions on who or what would be said or done on Fire Island. And the trips back on the L.I.R.R. were even more graphic in nature plotting our future office trysts and parties. Remember, this was the swag of the 70s.

But in the city, proper, we were the Kingpins of our indoor court on the higher rung of the corporate ladder. Our file clerk when first asked, "What's your name?" introduced himself to us nervously, because we were the Office Kings, as "Pablo,... uh, uh,... Pablo." So that became his name around the office. It was an office joke: "Pablo, Pablo." He was the Puerto Rican member accepted into our office men's club.

We were also the Kingpins of the outdoor courts. Regular basketball games were played on concrete while shooting at those chain nets in Chinatown. Those nets made a special clanking sound rather than the swish of rope nets. You all know those sounds that are etched into our street ball memories. It is hard to forget those sounds. Twelve Kingpins of all shapes and sizes regularly piled into an old Chevy to drive over to the courts. The games were tough. I mean I was a 'player' but there were some rocks I could not move in the post. Behemoths like Gerry, Jeff the Giant, and Joe were rough to battle with. These guys were not into fitness program routines, they were just strong! It was manly fun on Fridays after the work day was finished. One time we were playing on these same Chinatown courts. While looking up in horror we could see hundreds of high school age boys charging down the courts with fights spontaneously breaking out. Most of us steeled ourselves thinking we were the objects of gang turf claims. They passed us and continued the fight down the street as the New York City police closed in on them, maybe with 'stop and frisk' on their minds, the policy of law enforcement epitomized by the Michael Bloomberg administration in 2012 and 2013.[41]

Times have changed. I noticed it in the office at the turn of this century. I think this was the era of the dot-com bubble. The dot-com bubble (also known as the dot-com boom, the tech bubble, and the internet bubble) was a period of excessive investment speculation mainly in the United States that occurred roughly from 1994 to 2000, a period of extreme growth in the use and adoption of the internet.[42] [Conversations were no longer hosted by the coffee pot. Partitions were set up for work in cubicles. Office workers became isolated from one another.]

So on we marched into the advent of the personal computer and smart phone era. No longer do we even have to converse at the job. We have become shell creatures of what we once were. Just testing our endurance over the use of broad band width and knowing that we can be hacked by the Russians, our Facebook accounts are easy to hack into and the constitutional privacy protections are things of the past. Fake news and Twitter rants are the new normal. And so it is that many professionals turn to a welcome source of relief; bowing to the idols of the fitness gods. Let's join the health club!!

With the advent of social media, it is sad that today most people only lift their heads for a moment or two from that banal instrument of plastic and precious metals used to fuel smart phones. The rare earth metal dysprosium is

"They are rare earths, a group of 17 chemical elements with tongue-tying names such as yttrium and thulium that are used in televisions, cell phones, laptops, cars, cancer treatment drugs, nuclear reactor shields, aircraft engines, and weapons. Coveted for their magnetic and conductive properties, they make technologies faster, stronger, lighter, and more efficient. "Without rare earths and the miniaturization capabilities they provide, computers would be the size of classrooms instead of the size of smartphones," says Julie Michelle Klinger, an assistant professor of international relations at Boston University's Frederick S. Pardee School of Global Studies."[43]

just one example - Atomic number 66. Not only is it running low in availability since it does not run freely in nature (with shortages predicted to get problematic by 2020-ish) but its unique magnetic powers are also key in burgeoning green technologies like electric vehicles and wind turbines.

So now what are we to do? In the 21st century, violence is escalating and spiraling out of control exponentially, the world is warming in places we never thought possible to explore, our kids seem desensitized to what is going on around them in society. Pain killer addiction is reaching epic proportions. Somehow we have to find our way from all of this disconnect.

We need to create new new kinds of leadership, male or female, when faced with this new world order, or otherwise, the End Game for all of us will be reached sooner than civilization expects.

Chapter 10

Quirky Quests For Fitness Dreams
Observations At The Health Club

In some ways it is nice to have rediscovered the long lost art of conversation once held around the office coffee pot. I find it in the health club locker room as a way to reconnect with people.

Let's start with the introductory walk into the locker room at my health club.

Local health clubs can easily be a place to communicate with friends. Yes, you do hope that you will get healthy by going there but for many it is a "gossip" corner of today's world. It will provide you with myriad tales of ailments and 'trash talk' of many of it's members. Surgeries and surgeons are compared. Knee replacements, back and shoulder surgeries are very common. Men and women at the health club are worried about their own mortality.

There are a lot of people in pain. The elder statesman of our locker room group is Ed and he has been there since the club first opened. He thinks of himself, and is his best audience, as the alpha dog among men, so he will force himself to play racquetball several times a week despite the back and knee braces he has to wear. Afterwards you will find him slumped over the seats and aching in the hot tub. Even when it's a mere spittoon by Friday when they refill it, Ed will sit there no matter what. Splendidly jousting conversations are held with Ed on politics and education later as we explore the collegiality of the locker room.

We cling to these routines in order to stabilize our lives amidst the chaos we read or hear about. There are instances where club members cannot follow the routines for fitness because they have been "kicked out of class." Recently the locker room banter was about one of the trainers kicking Hal out of the class that he paid for! She said, "your form is no good, I'm tired of trying to teach you, you're not taking your training seriously, **NOW GET OUT!!**" Hal says this is like the detention he used to get in high school for misbehavior. The banter turned up the heat a notch when Joey, one of the other trainers, came into the locker and the guys were trying to sell him Hal as a client. "Hey, Joey, you wanna pick up another student? He's a good payer."

Hal owns the local shoe store and he fancies himself the expert on clothing etiquette. One day's lesson might be on socks. Hal says, in mimicry of former First Lady Michelle Obama when dressing yourself, you "go low and then come up high." That made sense to all of us. Then it went from the ridiculous to the sublime as he embellished on his story. He said always put your socks on first whether you are wearing shorts or pants and never wear short socks with jeans because it doesn't look good. I don't know what brand of socks he was talking about, and someone else yelled out, *"Yeah, Dumbass,* socks like on the radio and TV commercials." To add fuel to the fires of hilarity he started talking about some tight workout shorts that he had in his store with different colors. The guys called them Woo-Thongs and asked if they could get them in pink. Vinny, Dr. Vinny Boom Botz wanted to know if he could get them in flesh color and crotchless. You remember Dr. Vinny Boom Botz that

Rodney Dangerfield always spoke of so highly in his comedy routine. This guy Vinny has his huge toiletrie/medicine bag draped over his locker blocking the aisle. That's why we call him the Doctor. When he's in the pool he doesn't swim, he just does 'tippy-toe, tippy toe, like George Costanza's secret password in a Seinfeld episode. These are typical topics of locker room babel and, check this word out, katzenjammer.

Eda is another member of the Wet Team. She is 97 years young, and swimming at 5 a.m. each morning. She is a Holocaust victim but continues to follow her fitness routine.

Don is an advertising executive who knew the original club owner and he is the only member who has a 'lifetime membership.' That means he doesn't have to pay any dues. Some of the guys built him his own shelves in the lockers, he has four different lockers with all his clothes, towels sports equipment and toiletries sprawled out. I've never seen custom-made gym lockers before. We all kid him about how he should put us in his will for that 'lifetime membership.'

I have enough problems just getting an open locker. One thing I have to give Don credit for he will use his walker to get into the pool area, but once in the pool he does his laps like the rest of us. I commend him for this.

Sometimes I go to another aisle because I don't want to have to jump around guys who are taking up too much space. I then go to the next aisle and interfere with others and their fitness routines. I get an earful," Oh, you forgot which aisle you belong in, are you lost? You're lucky you weren't in here earlier it would have been standing room only." My retort was, "Hey, I just want to shake things up a bit for you guys, keep you on your tippy-toes" relishing my role as provocateur! This is their post-work-out and locker room banter and routine which they also follow religiously. Bonnie, Sam, Vinny, Eda, Don and all Wet Team members claim just being in the water invigorates them. Some of the swimmers hope to find the Fountain of Youth like the Spanish explorer, Ponce DeLeon.[44] For most of us the End Game is enjoying the pool and our fitness routines. It should not be the haunting words that Don repeats that "we are born to die." This, unfortunately, is his End Game. Hey, if he feels that way he should donate his 'lifetime' membership" and, of course, those lockers and shelves!

"The fact is that our lives are being transformed by the information age and now the genetic information age. We have mapped the human genome and now scientists can read and write DNA like software. George Church is the Harvard University scientist who has been using his own DNA as test samples.

"The fully assembled George Church is 6'5" and 65. He helped pioneer mapping the human genome and editing DNA. Today, his lab is working to make humans immune to all viruses, eliminate genetic diseases, and reverse the effects of time and aging." They are currently doing this editing in laboratory mice and spaniel dogs.

George says its "not really editing genes. It's the gene function which is going down, and so we're boosting it back up by putting in extra copies of the genes." The scope of human trials is at least 10 years away.

Church received donations from the Virgin Islands' foundation of deceased money manager and convicted sex offender Jeffrey Epstein. He says "you don't always know your donors as well as you would like, and I regret not knowing more about the donor." He added, "So-called tainted money can be used for good... like the tobacco money was used for good things. I certainly apologize for my poor awareness and judgment."[45]

Maybe some of these End Gamers should be watching *CBS 60 Minutes* so they get even more excited about extending our New Age immortality.[46]

Now returning to our more banal routines and trivialities of fitness which make up today's locker room antics. Jim, who we call "Tips" because of his wing tip shoes (he always has new shoes) brings his iPad® to the gym, his clothes are always pressed with dry cleaning labels and he has shoe trees for his shoes. Shoe trees!! I've never seen anyone ever have those in a gym before! He also parks his Mercedes® far away from any of the other cars in the parking lot. This is Tip's fitness routine. Oh, he says he retired as of December 31, but the pressed clothes for Tips are still hanging in the locker room. Old habits die hard!

Philly, who we call 'Philly the Flash,' has got more braces and pads than knees, wrists and ankles. He says he has a bad arthritic condition in his wrist but the doctor wants him to take some prescription drug where the side effects which include possible liver damage seem worse than the ailment he is attempting to cure. How many times have you seen this type of advertisement on TV? Big Pharma will help your memory loss, increase your sex drive, stabilize your heart condition, etc.

Old Man Buddy shows up everyday pulling his suitcase on wheels. He slowly deposits the cart on one side of the pool and then lumbers over to the other side of the pool where he even more slowly places his towel down. You have got to see this to believe it. He does his laps in snail-like fashion, and swims for at least an hour each day. Even his wall-turns on the laps are as slow as pouring cold maple syrup on top of a hot stack of pancakes. He will not be deterred in his game, though, no matter what! It is his fitness routine. Hey, he just wore a new red pair of swim trunks! He says, after 10 years with the same trunks it was about time to change them. We all agree with that assessment.

Bonnie sends text messages every day saying she is going crazy trying to sell her house and move away to Florida. She is a ranking member of the group and the most vivacious, keeping us all together for parties and willing to gossip on any topic that comes up. We will miss her when she moves but she's lucky she gets to swim in warm weather every day now.

Oscar is still trying to lose that famous

10 lbs. I have been hearing that tale of 'woe' for months. He must announce everyday his weight gain or loss after getting on the scale. Today, he played racquetball and swam and claims he lost 4 pounds. Other guys rush up and say "hold that scale for me!" He says he played Davey, the guy he describes as "the guy who wears knee braces and has grey hair." I said, "I don't know him but that basically describes everyone in here." But he also admits to eating an apple pie over a few days and is still eating those pastrami, chopped chicken liver and rye bread sandwiches late at night which is not helping his metabolism. You better keep playing racquetball son.

Jimmy is 5 foot, 4 inches but in pretty good shape. I regale him and the other guys with 70s Kingpin stories about Glen, the Delaware Midget, and Jeff, the Giant. We used to always say Glen had a big head. It was rumored that when one of us bought a suit, Glen could use the trimmings for a new suit for himself. In addition, we said "his head was so big when he buys a new hat he could throw the hat away and wear the box." Since Glen also had a summer home in Delaware, he was always bragging about how we gave him the moniker the Delaware Midget.

Jimmy, the other day misplaced his size 6 1/2 baby blue clog shower shoes with the holes in them. He bought them at either Hal's shoe store or in Amsterdam because they look like they come from Holland. They are really funny looking. He was tearing up the locker room looking for them. We all said that they looked like the midget submarines we used to get in the cereal boxes. For all of us it was lucky they were in the Lost and Found or we would never heard the end of who stole them. The guys said that one of the little kids might have taken them because they fit him perfectly.

Another legend the guys liked was Jeff who we called The Giant. He was 6 foot 4 inches tall, and he is the only person who I have heard of who had his rental car repossessed while gambling in Los Vegas casinos. We were supposed to go to Lake Mead and when we got outside the car was gone. He was seen going around the casino trying to borrow money. You know the saying "What happens in Vegas stays in Vegas" Not true. This story has now found it's way back to the health club and became part of our locker room legends.

We have our own creature references in the locker room. Max, is called "Creature" or Skate because he makes creature sounds but he can glide when he dances at the Club parties. He is always blowing his nose, clearing his throat and has a big creature-like 'fro' on his head. We kid him and say he still thinks he's a 70s Kingpin.

Then there is Joe, who I call Smiley because he only says he is happy when he finishes his workout. Never before and he, especially hates the Christmas and New Year holidays. You can't talk to Smiley before he ts working out because he is, absolutely, never in a good mood. He works at the Golf Course and has stories about those crazy, rich Asians who don't follow the Club rules because they talk too much in groups and hold up the entire course. He has to go out there frequently and 'shoo' them along the way.

Smiley says, just like Comedian Ronny Chieng on Netflix' *Destroying America,* that these are rich, crazy Asians and golf to them with their fancy cloth covers on their drivers, woods and irons represents prestige. Being a club member means wealth. He says these are the top two criteria for Asian doctors whose parents have pushed them into that career. He says caring for their patients is low on the

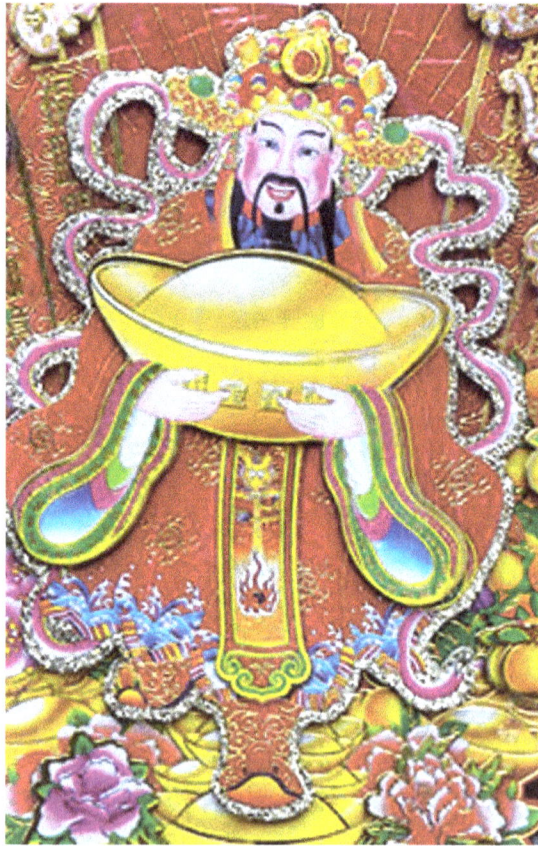

Art from paper lucky charm found in Bangkok. Artist unknown.

Legend says that every lunar New Year, Ts'ai Shen, the God of Wealth, descends from heaven to inspect his followers. This is the Year of the Rat, my year, so I am very Happy. Many families worship the God of Wealth in the early morning, by offering incense and invite the god into their homes. Chinese people will eat dumplings or dim sum on this day, as they are thought to resemble ancient gold.

People say that after being offered sacrifices, Ts'ai Shen leaves for heaven on the second day of the lunar New Year. People will burn the picture they welcomed on the New Year's Eve and see the deity off, wishing for a luckier and more prosperous year. So everyone buy my book on LOCKER TALES AND FITNESS!

priority list. This defines for them what makes for success in America. The Asians even have a god of money which they worship, Ts'ai Shen, the god of wealth.[47] Ts'ai Shen, also called Cai Boxing Jun, in the Chinese religion, the popular god (or gods) of wealth, widely believed to bestow on his devotees the riches carried about by his attendants. During the two-week New Year celebration, incense is burned in Caishen's temple (especially on the fifth day of the first lunar month), and friends joyously exchange the traditional New Year greeting "May you become rich" ("Gongxi facai").

So, Smiley must have had his hands really full on this one, wouldn't you say? " Ronny says what we need in America is an Asian president to negotiate between the races because Asians don't care for one side or another. They are neutral. They would be analytical in solving problems like: deficit spending, global warming, separation of powers, and impeachment. They have good math skills. Just give them a week, problem solved! It is an ironic suggestion because in 1882 the U. S. Congress passed the Chinese Exclusionary Act, kicking Chinese out of the country after they helped build the Trans-Continental Railroad. Revisiting

Andrew Yang, for president, maybe??

Despite these personal quirks and verbal joustings, which add humor in the locker room, most of these gym rats don't stray too far from the big picture of End Game immortality which goes on in our modern era. I suspect they are all trying to stay the aging process. One example of striving to reach this End Game is the story of cryogenics.[48,49] Robert Ettinger and Bob Nelsons' efforts in the 1960s aimed at preserving people in a state of suspended animation so they could wake up in the future and be cured of their ailments.

Ted Williams, the Hall of Fame baseball player of the Boston Red Sox willed that this be done with his body in the hopes of a future cure. After Williams died on July 5, 2002, his body was taken by private jet to a company in Scottsdale, Arizona. There, Williams's body was separated from his head in a procedure called neuroseparation, according to the magazine.[50]

The operation was complete and Williams's head and body were preserved separately. The head is stored in a steel can filled with liquid nitrogen. It had been shaved, drilled with holes and accidentally cracked ten times, the magazine said. Williams's body stands upright in a 9-foot tall cylindrical steel tank, also filled with liquid nitrogen. So, theoretically, and I only say this tongue-in-cheek, if Williams's head were placed on another man's body, he might wake up one day in the future and say "I can see it but I can't hit it!" He was known as the "Kid" and also the "Splendid Splinter" – thin as a rail and splendid with the bat. I actually visited Fenway Park in Boston last fall and saw the seat which is specially marked in red with the number "502" the distance his home run traveled into right field and no one has ever since hit one that far. He hit a man's straw hat, Joseph Boucher, and knocked it off. It is Section 42, Row 37 seat 21.[51]

In the movie, *The Avengers-End Game,* also out in 2019, the movie is attempting to further our education about suspended animation. Capt. America, Steve Rogers, who had been frozen for 70 years comes out of suspended animation to fight the End Game against Thanos. How does he survive being under ice for all that time?[52]

So from a scientific perspective what exactly is this 'suspended animation'? Is it just another mysterious fantastical term that's far from the realm of the physical world (which many of us may crave)... or is it something real?

Suspended Animation

Yes, suspended animation is a real thing!

To give you a quick definition, suspended animation is the slowing down, or altogether stopping, of certain life processes through certain means without causing the death of the person in question.

The concept of suspended animation has been discussed several times in fiction; page opposite is an 1852 depiction of Snow White laid in a glass coffin during her period of magic-induced suspended animation.

Involuntary bodily processes, such as our heartbeat and breathing, may occur, but you would need artificial means to detect them. In fact, very small organisms (such as embryos of up to eight cells) are preserved in this way, and some have been kept in preservation for as long as 13 years!

Such a suspended state of living can be induced using certain methods, including temperature alterations and chemical changes. It has been seen that lowering the temperature

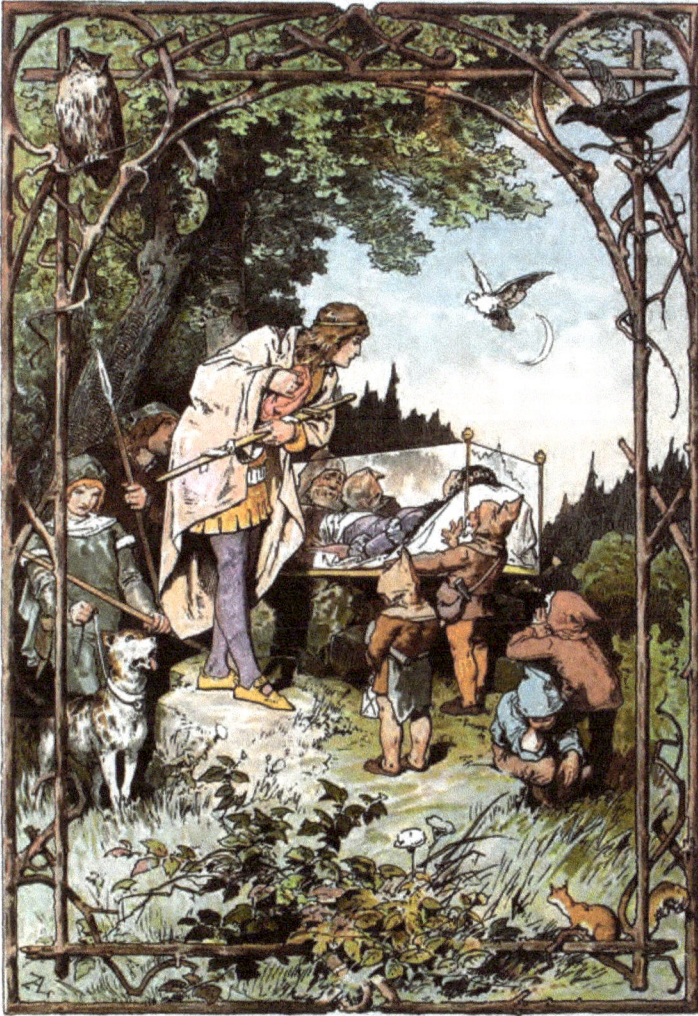

ARTIST: Darstellung von Alexander Zick (1845-1907), for Grimm's Fairy Tales, late 1800s.

Snow White and Suspended Animation.
Schneewittchen ('Snow White' in German)

of a substance lowers its 'chemical activities' (Arrhenius equation). Metabolism, an incredibly vital chemical activity that occurs within the human body, falls under such 'chemical activities'. It has a long way to go!

It will be many years before we can send astronauts to distant destinations using suspended animation.

Such a process, as of now, is far more complex than what they showed in *Captain America*. A human body cannot survive, even in a state of suspended animation, while being exposed to excessive cold temperatures for such long periods of time. There are simply too many pitfalls involved, including damage from ice formation and the loss of cellular viability, not to mention the ethical ramifications of freezing someone in such inhospitable conditions. With all these roadblocks, a distinct lack of experimentation limits our chances of understanding it much further.

Presently, we need to be better equipped, both in terms of understanding the process and technological know-how, to be able to recreate anything close to the super-heroic survival of *Captain America*.

As it turns out, surviving for extended periods of time in extremely cold temperatures IS possible, but getting your hands on super-soldier serum and vita rays... not so much.[53]

Suggested Reading:
The Courageous Captain America.[54]

Chapter 11

Collegiality and Fitness in the Locker Room

B ut the history of fitness didn't really begin until the 1970s. Prior to 1970, blue-collar workers held the majority of jobs in America. For this working class, manual labor was a normal part of everyday life. Pushing, pulling, lifting, carrying, running and a wide variety of physical tasks were part of a typical workday. Exercising (or participating in physical activity to develop or maintain fitness) wasn't necessary. In fact, back in the 1970s, only 24 percent of adults reported exercising routinely. It wasn't until after the 1970s that Americans (primarily white-collar, middle class workers) began exercising on a regular basis. For this generation, work demands shifted from manual labor to office work requiring very little physical effort and the workday consisted of sitting idle at a work desk. [In fact, today if you look at many of the job descriptions listed on *Indeed* or *Glassdoor*, the job requirements include the ability to lift anywhere from 20-50 lbs., which I am sure were not previously part of job qualifications prior to the 1970s since it was a presumption.]

Over the next two decades the idea of a "physical elite", an exclusive group of very active and fit human beings who exercised regularly (if not excessively), ate very clean and healthy, were self-aware and incredibly successful in their upper-middle income bracket jobs spurred the memberships of numerous country clubs and private social clubs across the country. It was, in essence, the idea of a "super race" committed to achieving the perfect body and mind through exercise and good nutrition.

As a result, participation in running groups and private clubs grew at unprecedented rates. One needs to just look at the number of marathon participants in New York as an example where the numbers have increased from 127 in 1972 to a record of over 52,000 in 2018. Staggering numbers as the fitness craze has exponentially increased in 50 years time. In addition, by 1987, a nationwide Gallup poll revealed 69 percent of Americans reported exercising regularly.

Time Magazine reported in its November 7, 2019, issue that even if we run less because of restrictions on time, we should at least get in 50 minutes per week of cardio work. The analysis is the latest to illustrate the benefits of running on the human body. "It's what we evolved to do," says Daniel Lieberman, a professor of human evolutionary biology at Harvard University (who was not involved in the new research). People may no longer chase down prey for their next meal, but running is still helping us survive: as leisure-time exercise, it keeps us healthy." One of the best ways to avoid having to see a doctor," Lieberman says, "is to stay physically active."[55]

Just this weekend I was walking on the river path and I found a cell phone. When I called the number it tracked and someone called us back. Apparently, daughter-marathoner's Pop-Pop while riding his bike and trying to keep up with the runners dropped his cellphone three times while daughter was off running her marathon. He told me a car ran over the phone one time. Hey, at least Pop-Pop is getting in his cardio work.

Although commercial fitness centers have been around since the 1940's, the emergence of the modern fitness center was driven by cultural changes that shaped the industry we see today. Attitudes towards health and wellness (or more accurately, obesity and associated preventable disease) fuel the continuous growth of the industry, affecting the habits and expectations of three generations of Americans and beyond.

Several cultural changes contributed to the fitness movement, including:

☞ The desire to be healthy
☞ The desire to "fit in"
☞ Corporate expectations and culture
☞ The changing roles of women
☞ The media[56]

Let us analyze each of these elements as it relates to current day health club climate.

Those of us, mere mortals, have to be satisfied with the work we do to fight against the elements of our body's attrition. My friend, Oscar wears his favorite cowboy hat and calls himself Tex. He will drive hours to go skiing upstate New York or hoist his bike down to the Jersey shore to pedal along the boardwalk. Then he gains back the 10 lbs. from his End Game, by hoisting up a flask of brandy while sitting on the beach.

Ed wears a back brace and knee pads but continues to play racquetball even if it kills him and, who knows, it just might. Look at 51 year old Joe Morrison, flanker back of the New York Giants football team in the 1960s. A strenuous game of racquetball did in 'Old Dependable.'[57]

I have already mentioned Eda and our daily swims and how they form a part of our immortality dreams. Joining us are other members of the Wet Team like Bonnie, Old Man Buddy and Veronica who swim constantly even when they are on vacation. Don only swims on Sundays and that is his end game of enjoyment. I give Veronica a lot of credit because she is in the pool at 5 a.m. with Eda and in a machine-like fashion churns through the water prior to heading out to her job. This is a rain, snow or fair weather event. All of these efforts are to insure that we meet the first criteria of being healthy.

There are small training groups of 3-5 persons every morning at the health club ting at 5:00 a.m., jumping off stations with medicine balls, twirling long ropes, and the use of machines for toning up the muscles. Maybe it's the early morning hour but I don't observe a whole lot of collegiality around these sessions. This is serious stuff going on there. This may be a factor of rushing for time in the workday or just seeing fitness as the End Game of life. There is a cadre of trainers who assist you in working on specific exercises. I think you have to be a certified physical trainer to do this job from the National Academy of Sports Medicine but your livelihood is directly proportional to how many persons you can sign up for the training. I always feel the probing eyes of the trainers seeking to scoop up new clients as I sometimes drop in for a mild work-out on the machines. So a cottage industry of fitness trainers has grown alongside the desire to be healthy and immortal.

Many immigrants to our country have seen fitness and athletics as way of fitting in to American culture so that they will not be outliers. This is our next criteria, the desire to fit in. There are other athletes from other countries who exemplify the style of discipline and perseverance in keeping fit. Marty Glickman was the famed Knicks and football Giant sportscaster of the 1960s. I remember driving in the car with my family and listening to his broadcasts of the New York Giants football team with Al DiRogatis. He was the second fastest sprinter in the United States in competition for the U.S. Olympic team in 1936. He and Sam Stoller did not run their event at the Games because they were Jewish and the President of the Olympic Committee, Avery Brundage did not want to insult Adolf Hitler. Glickman to his dying day regretted not running at the Games. Glickman was born in the Bronx, New York, to a Romanian Jewish family. His parents, Harry and Molly Glickmann, had migrated to the United States from Iaşi, Romania.[58]

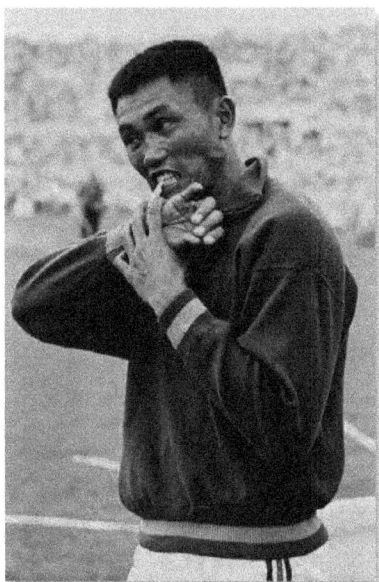

Yang Chuan-kwang (C.K. Yang) at the 1960 Olympics.

I remember my fascination with C.K. Yang of Taiwan who was in second place going into the 1960 Olympics to Rafer Johnson. He was so much smaller and yet he was indomitable.

Chuan-kwang at the 1960 Olympics was in second place going into the final event of the decathalon, the 1500 meter run, Yang trailed Johnson by just 67 points, but Johnson hung on to win the gold medal, with Yang placing second. Yang topped Johnson in all four track events and three jumping or vaulting events, but Johnson gained a large margin in the three throwing events (the shot put, the discus throw, and the javelin throw). Yang was the first Olympic medallist in his country's history.[59]

I also followed the career of Jeremy Lin in the NBA whose Taiwanese family supported him as he persisted in his devotion to the game, which led to his spectacular 2012 'Linsanity' run with the New York Knicks including a 38 point performance against Kobe Bryant and the L.A. Lakers. I still have his Linsanity tee shirt!! He just practiced hard, stayed fit and met the challenges that were thrown against him. Seven years after "Linsanity" took over the N.B.A., and months after he became the first Asian-American player to win a championship ring, Jeremy Lin has signed with the Beijing Shougang Ducks of the Chinese Basketball Association, the team announced on Tuesday.

There was a chilly N.B.A. free agency market for Lin, 31, who split last season between the Atlanta Hawks and Toronto Raptors. He played only 27 minutes for the Raptors in the playoffs, including just one mop-up minute in the finals.

J Lin has always been about more than just basketball. Years from now, I'm sure we'll hear even more about the difficulties he faced in being one of the first Asian-Americans in the modern era to play in the NBA.

In the meantime, we'll continue to follow his career in China. And, who knows, there may be another opportunity in the NBA before he hangs up his sneakers and calls it a career.[60]

Michael Chang's family is also from Taiwan. He is the youngest male player in history to win a Grand Slam tennis event, winning the 1989 French Open at 17 years and 95 days old Chang won a total of 34 top-level professional singles titles, was a three-time Grand Slam tennis event runner-up, and reached a career-best ranking of world No. 2 in 1996. Since he was shorter than virtually all of his opponents, he played a dogged defensive style utilizing his quickness and speed.[61]

Let's not forget Michelle Kwan, who rose to prominence in figure skating, winning five World titles and capturing medals at two Olympic Games. Her family emigrated from Canton, PRC and Hong Kong, but had to scrape by financially to support Michelle from the age of five in her persistence and devotion to skating.[62]

When I joined the club I also was an outlier. I knew nobody and nobody appeared to want to know who I was. Gradually between the grunts and groans of the exercise routines, I became a daily visitor who was accepted. Even while swimming laps, I will throw those plastic floating noodles and rubber duckies into Sam and Bonnie's lap lanes. I enjoyed bringing some levity and breaking up the serious aspects of their training routines. But a lot of times the conversations come around to who had bad knees, a bad back or has problems with arthritis?

One of the points of levity is "The Legend of Scuba Steve." We joke around and call Oscar Scuba Steve because just like in the movie, *Big Daddy*, Sam likes to come to the pool with his flippers, weights on his arms, radio with music to swim by, goggles, silicone ear plugs, etc. Then he typically leaves this bag of stuff behind at the pool. The rest of the Wet Team, have to bring the stuff to him. "Hey Scuba Steve, you're like a middle schooler leaving his stuff all around. This is not *Pee Wee's Playhouse* here!!"

Now I am privileged to be part of the locker room guy-talk. Ronnie says as part of his fitness routine that "I got to do the banana roll or the banana crunch" To which I reply "that only makes me more hungry for breakfast." Ronnie is one of the good guys in the locker room but he, like many, say he doesn't care about the politicking just whether his 401(K) has gone up. Now, in light of the coronavirus scare, the market and his 401(K) are tanking in value. He does not appear to be as satisfied with the Trump administration's handling of the crisis and the economy. Even though I have strong differences of opinion on many issues with other members of the locker room and Hot Tub Kingpins and the *#Push-Back Brigade* the politicking and collegiality continues to go on at the club. We don't take each other too seriously.

Now here comes the Politicking!

Like I previously mentioned, Ed who sits religiously in that spittoon of a hot tub, will argue with you over the merits of the Trump election victory in 2016. For some impervious reason Ed does not feel that Mr. Trump is legally required to disclose his tax returns. [Lo and behold, on October 11, 2019, the U.S. Circuit Court of Appeals reaffirmed the District Court of New York's decision that President Trump must hand over 8 years of tax returns which have been subpoenaed by Cyrus Vance's New York District Attorney's office.][63]

The President still claims, even though impeached, that there is nothing to the whistle-blower complaint which alleges President Trump made the supposed call on July 25 to UkrainianPresident Volodymyr Zelensky telling him, "if you could look into it," to work with his personal attorney, Rudolph Giuliani and U.S. Attorney General William P. Barr to investigate the conduct of Democratic presidential candidate Joe Biden and his family in the Ukraine and threatening the withdrawal of close to 400 million dollars in much needed aid to the Ukraine if he did not comply.[64] We of the Hot Tub Kingpins are seeking the answer to the burning question of what is a *Quid Pro Quo?*

The basic concept behind *"quid pro quo"* can be summed up in a more colloquial saying in English: If you scratch my back, I'll scratch yours.

Of course, I cite Mick Mulvaney, White

House acting chief of staff, and his squishy, sushi-like flip-flop, on again-off again testimony on the now famous Ukraine phone call.[65] Talking about flip-flops we also have Ambassador Gordon Sondland, a political appointee by President Trump, and not at all a career diplomat who suddenly found his memory and now

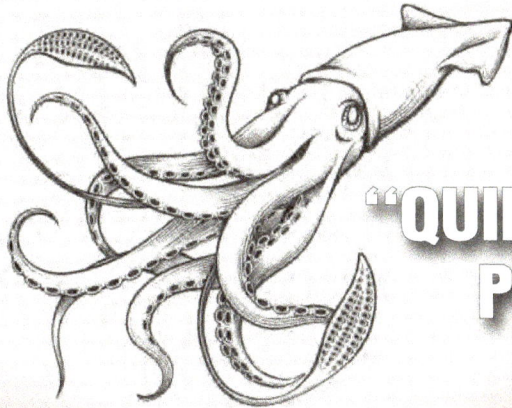

DO YOU KNOW:
The Defintion of

"QUID PRO QUO"

IMAGE: © Can Stock Photo / Olena1983

A. *Legal accountability*
B. *A contentious work environment*
C. *Something for something*
D. *Tasty sushi made from squid*
E. *None of the above*

Of coulrse, if you'll remember your *Latin* from high school, or from your law school days, the correct answer is C, "something for something."

states that there definitely was a *quid pro quo* with Ukraine over obtaining their foreign aid in exchange for investigating the Biden family in their country.[66]

President Trump says we are "kicking their 'ass' on this impeachment inquiry[67] as we await the actual beginnings of the public proceedings. My buddies Ed and Sam respond that this *quid pro quo* is just foreign policy as usual. "No quid without the quo" they say.

This whistleblower complaint prompted the Democrats to commence an impeachment inquiry and judiciary committee hearings on the threats, abuse of Presidential authority and 'high crimes and misdemeanors such as bribery' and attempts to cover these threats up. The fruits of this inquiry are touched on in satirical skits by Alec Baldwin and the cast of *Saturday Night Live*, and this issue will continue to be explored over the next few months by the press all prior to the 2020 election. President Trump's response was to say "this whistleblower and colleagues are like spies and traitors." Speaking to the United States Mission to the United Nations the President said, "you know what we used to do with these people back in the old days?"[68] Better yet, let's hang, draw and quarter these traitors, as they did in the Middle Ages!"[69] But of course for us this is all about collegiality in the locker room.

We are sometimes joined in the hot tub by Sam, our very own "Oscar," the retired Wall Street trader, now slicing bologna in the deli, who thinks that the economy is doing just grand. I don't think the market surge is putting more money in his pockets and this is what puzzles me. How can these guys profess their loyalty to the Trump administration even when

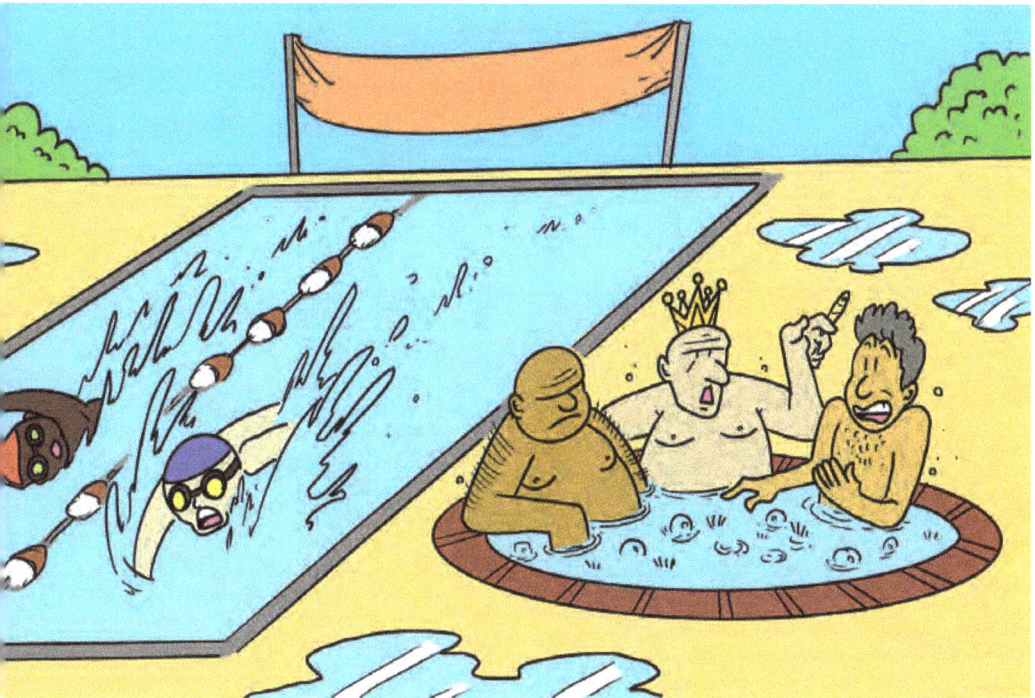

Politiking and congeniality in the hot tub but 'keeping it real.'

they are not benefiting from his policies. GM went on strike for three weeks, oh well, as GM goes so goes the country. But of course I am all for collegiality in the locker room!

President Trump doesn't believe there is anything in science that can prove global warming, despite the mass protest rallies of young people pointing to their future on this planet. But it does provide us with the grist mill for the hot tub and, as I walk into the locker room, a cry goes out "Hey, here comes the Democrat!!" Karl chimes in as he has my back when it comes to President Trump, "Just follow the rouble." Now with the impeachment inquiry it is more likely to be, "Follow the Ukrainian hryvnia."

More recently we have the testimony of Ambassador William Taylor, the senior U.S. diplomat in the Ukraine who has unequivocally testified before impeachment investigators that he was told the release of military aid to Kiev was contingent on a public declaration that Ukraine would investigate the Bidens and the 2016 election and he felt that this was just "crazy to demand."[70]

Post-Script and News Flash:

President Trump returns to New York to attend the UFC matches,[71] but on Halloween declares Florida to be his residence and Governor Andrew Cuomo says to Florida, "Good riddance, Take him he doesn't pay his taxes anyway!"[72]

And guess what - The Trump Beat Goes On.

These interactions for me definitely replace those held around the office coffee pot of the 70s. I accept the changes in the Kingdom. But, remember again, this is all about collegiality in the locker room!

The next criteria for fitness is that of the corporate structure and culture. Corporations today require that their personnel be physically fit and able to work long hours in the workday.

They provide gyms within the corporate headquarters so less time can be spent away from work with more time being devoted to office matters. This is a shortening of the leisure time in the day and as more emphasis is put on the workforce to conform to the rigors of the corporate culture there is less down time for individuals to socialize. In addition, in just the opposite way, because of the advent of the personal computer more people are working from home and have less interaction there with fellow employees necessitating the need to join or have personal gyms. In either instance though, the modern day fitness routine is an offshoot of corporate culture.

With the advancement of women into the workplace, the next criteria shows that women wish to keep themselves physically attractive for the rigors of the job and to achieve higher ranking status within the corporate structure. The glass ceiling has cracks that have developed in it, if not totally smashed. There is more emphasis for women on job status and less on their office relationships. More women are participating in fitness programs. In my club, I do not see a lot of interaction between men and women as everyone seems to be concentrating solely on their exercise regime at least, those who are conforming to a work schedule and are very goal-oriented in their fitness training and performance.

It is easy to understand that the retired members have an obviously more leisurely and relaxed approach to their exercise routines. This approach to fitness is maybe something that the club and its membership can incorporate in the future. I definitely say that some of our 65+ year old swimmers are really very healthy and in terrific shape. So it can pay dividends to approach our road to fitness as an end game, not the ultimate End Game of those fixated on the rigidity of their fitness routines and mortality.

The next criteria of fitness is social media which does play an important part in the fitness industry. You can see YouTube videos espousing fitness programs as well as TV and newspaper advertisements for personal trainers. I noticed that in the local movie theaters' ads for the local fitness clubs as well. The health club where I belong has a monthly newsletter, a website for its members and also text messages about upcoming programs. What this does is incorporate issues of fitness more into our daily lives so that one cannot remove themselves from its impact. The clubs in the community compete against each other for subscriptions, each one offering a different set of membership criteria and pricing.

Where and when will it end? I don't know the answer to that question. As previously mentioned and even up to the post-World War II era our ancestors didn't worry about these daily exercise programs or being afflicted by ailments.

The knights of President Trump's America seek to champion their conquest of Iran and the modern day Levant. The knights of the Middle Ages would continue to press for more land and control of Jerusalem as they sought survival and were not dependent and in contemplation of their own mortality.

In the post-World War eras, it is informative to note that families' primary concern was more about making a living in the modern world and utilizing the G.I. bill to buy that little house with the picket fence. "Get your cat off my lawn," Tony Aiello says to Anthony LaPaglia, while watering his Kentucky Bluegrass. "The heat of his body is burning a hole in my grass." This was the most important thing to the man of the house in the 1960s. See the 1991 movie, *29th Street*.

American soldiers and cowboys in the 19th and 20th centuries expanded American influence and power in the world. Programs of structured fitness would have been a non-sequitur to them. Rather they just hoisted up a cup of 'six shooter'[73] coffee which was strong and black and slogged out onto the range. This was more likely their rallying cry.

I wonder as I get more and more middle

of the night tweets and an onslaught of comments on social issues or sporting events whether our consumption of stimulants (such as coffee or opioids) or our routines of programmed fitness are making us more stressed out and subjecting modern man to even more extreme burn out. In our quest to run more marathons, sell more real estate, day trade as many stocks in our portfolio are we doing more damage to ourselves and the world around us? The questions remain and I am sure will be explored in the years to come.

I am reminded of the Inuit Canadian ranger, Marvin Atqittuq, who said "We Inuit have been talking about this climate change stuff for a long time and now the government wants us to keep a lookout," Marvin's 74 year old father, Jacob's response to the author's frozen facial burn at Lake Kakivakturvik in the Arctic region, pressing his thumb to the burn he said 'good.' I think he meant not so bad. "Jacob had been born in an igloo and survived brutal winters and hungry bears, searing frostbite, boat accidents and a season of famine which killed many Inuit. Each morning he woke before us, and at the foot of the mattress we all shared, he cooked bannock, a sweet, doughy bread, and softly sang old church hymns in Inuktitut."[74,75] I wonder if modern man in his present state of fitness could do the same as Jacob Atqittuq.

I still remain, however, a kindred soul hoping to aid and educate for the future of humanity When it comes to winning at life and the fitness game it goes like this:

"Sometimes when you win, you really lose, and sometimes when you lose, you really win, and sometimes when you win or lose, you actually tie, and sometimes when you tie, you actually win or lose. Winning or losing is all one big organic globule, from which one extracts what one needs."

— Gloria Clement (Rosie Perez), in 1992 movie ***White Men Can't Jump***, written by Ron Sheldon.

EXTRACT WHAT YOU NEED FROM THE ROADMAP TO FITNESS

A Cacophony of Collegiality and Politicking

The Locker Room Boys continue the debate and add more fuel for the Hot Tub Kingpins
The weeks of November 11-18, 2019

⭐ The New York Second Circuit Court of Appeals ruled on Nov. 4th President Trump must turn over 8 years of tax returns setting the stage for a 'Supreme Court Clash' [76]

⭐ The financial records of Deutsche Bank, President Trump's personal bank, were subponead by Congress, which case is likely to be heard by the U.S. Supreme Court. [77]

⭐ In defense of the subpoenas issued to him by Manhattan District Attorney, Cyrus R. Vance, Jr., Mr. Trump's attorneys had argued that his executive privilege and immunity from suit means he could literally 'walk down Fifth Avenue and shoot someone and not be held liable.' [78]

⭐ It is speculated that Mr. Trump's residence and domicile change to Florida is intended to avoid having to respond to the subpoenas previously issued. [79]

⭐ In regard to the ongoing crisis of the California wild fires and the potential federal budget shutdown on November 21, President Trump threatened to cut off FEMA aid for

for wildlife fire recovery efforts. "Unless they get their act together, which is unlikely, I have ordered FEMA to send no more money. It is a disgraceful situation in lives and money."[80]

⭐ Mexican drug dealers are sawing through President Trump's wall and creating holes large enough for adults to go through. They are also using step ladders to go over the wall. President Trump was quoted as saying it is virtually impenetrable and likening the structure to a Rolls-Royce.®[81]

⭐ While giving her testimony, before the House Intelligence Committee on November 15, 2019, Ambassador Marie Yvanovitch and the Committee receive President Trump's tweet in real time that she is 'bad news' and has been bad as an ambassador going back to her posting in Mogadishu and Somalia. This could potentially have been another impeachment grounds, besides that of bribery and high crimes and misdemeanors, of witness tampering and intimidation, and would have a chilling effect on witnesses coming forward.[82]

✪ Roger Stone, a highly thought of Trump ally, is convicted by a jury of perjuring himself over lying about his status as an intermediary of information from Wikileaks and the release of hacked Hillary Clinton emails. In September, 2017, in testimony before the House Intelligence Committee, Stone downplayed his ties to WikiLeaks. He was also convicted of witness tampering and intimidation. And, importantly, he claimed he had exchanged no emails, texts, or documents of any kind related to WikiLeaks or its founder, Julian Assange. Stone also said that he did not communicate with the Trump campaign about what he claimed to have learned about the WikiLeaks' plans to release emails. He faced up to 20 years in prison.[83]

✪ One thing for sure, President Trump wants his own live TV show after his days in the White House are over.

He wants to call it *The Apprentice-White House*, but it would more aptly be called *"The Never Trumper Show."* It could easily be modeled on Festivus. Festivus is a holiday held on December 23, where everyone complains to an unadorned aluminum pole

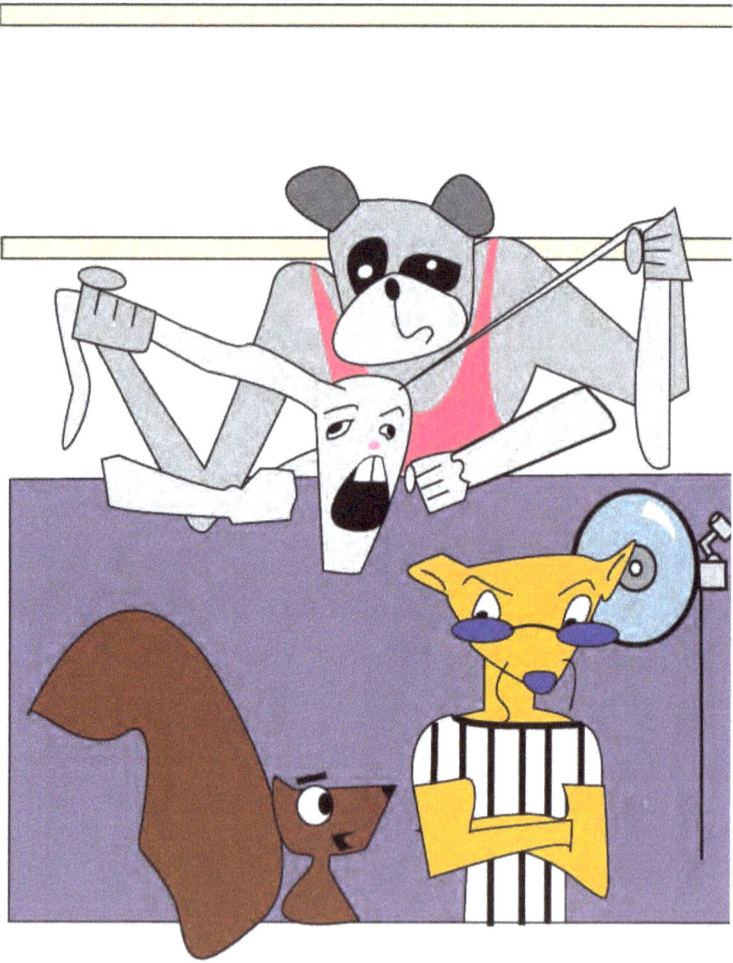

ARTIST: Peter Campbell

"The Never Trumper Show"

about someone or something, which is called an airing of grievances.

The culminating activity is where the head of the household, in this case it would be President Trump, selects one person at the Festivus celebration and challenges them to a feat of strength like a wrestling match.[84]

A PRIMER ON THE TRUMP IMPEACHMENT

⭐ "Ambassador to the EU, Gordon Sondland told Trump that Zelensky 'loves your ass.'" David Holmes, a State Department official, wrote in his opening statement, "[I then heard over the phone and rather loudly] President Trump ask, 'So, he's gonna do the investigation?' Ambassador Sondland replied that 'he's gonna do it,' adding that President Volodymyr Zelensky will do 'anything you ask him to.'" Holmes also writes that he asked Sondland if it was true that the president doesn't "give a s--- about Ukraine." Sondland, according to Holmes, confirmed this and said that Trump only cares about "big stuff," which was later defined as, 'big stuff' that benefits the President, like the Biden investigation that Mr. Giuliani was pushing."[85] "Not the war with Russia in the Ukraine?" Holmes asked.

⭐ President Trump complained of chest pains and is driven to Walter Reed Hospital, not flown. A separate source familiar with the situation described Trump's visit as "abnormal," but added that Trump, 73, appeared to be in good health late Friday. Some speculate this to be a ruse to avoid impeachment, laying the foundation for not running in 2020 and being pardoned by Vice-President Mike Pence.[86]

✪ Colonel Alexander Vindman, who did serve as the Director for European Affairs at the National Security Council, stands up in full military uniform, to the questioning of Rep. Jim Jordan, (R-OH) the man who never wears a suit and is always in 'attack mode' wearing his blue shirt sleeves began his line of rigorous questioning as to whether his colleagues and boss questioned his "judgment," and whether he leaked information [you have to remember that he was specifically placed on the investigation committee for his aggressive nature of cross-examination]. Jordan read from the deposition of Tim Morrison, Vindman's boss at the National Security Council, in which Morrison expressed "concerns" about Vindman's "judgment." Fiona Hill, another NSC official who also served as Vindman's boss, also had reservations – according to Jordan. "Your colleagues had concerns about your judgment. And your colleagues felt that there were times when you leaked information. Any idea why they have those impressions, Colonel Vindman?" Jordan asked. Vindman's reply was to read from his service evaluations for exercising excellent judgment as a government service employee.

Vindman added, "I can't say why Mr. Morrison questioned my judgment. We had only recently started working together. "And colonel, you never leaked information?," Jordan interjected.

"I never did, I never would," Vindman said. "That is preposterous that I would do that."[87]

⭐ In his testimony on Wednesday, November 20, 2019, Ambassador to the European Union Gordon Sondland threw Rudy Giuliani, and by implication, President Trump 'under the bus'. Giuliani's actions were characterized as inappropriately meddling in foreign policy and that he also mentioned that a number of top officials in President Donald Trump's administration were complicit in Giuliani's pursuit of a *"quid pro quo"* from Ukrainian President Volodymyr Zelensky. In one striking moment from his testimony, Sondland made clear that Secretary of State Mike

Pompeo was not only deeply involved in Giuliani's escapades but that he continued to involve Giuliani, the president's personal attorney, in State Department matters even after a whistleblower raised concerns. "They were all in the Loop."[88,89]

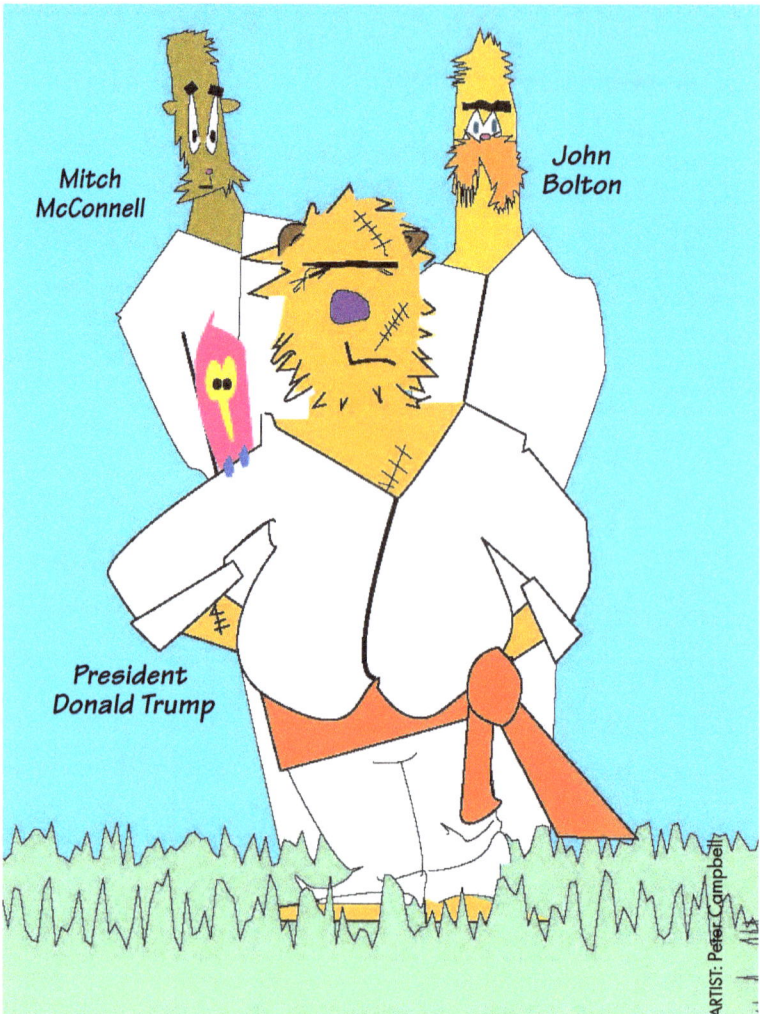

The Impeachment Trial

⭐ After the Sondland testimony President Trump declares that as to the phone conversation and what he was requesting of Zalensky on July 26, "I WANT NOTHING, I WANT NOTHING, NO QUID PRO QUO, TELL ZELENSKY TO DO THE RIGHT THING!!"[90]

⭐ Doesn't this sound similar to Sergeant Schultz on the 60s and 70s TV show *Hogan's Heroes*, – " I hear nothing, I see nothing?"

⭐ Now we heard all along that NSA Chief, John Bolton, may speak to his perceptions on the "Giuliani Drug Deal" in the Ukraine which led to the pressure on President Zalensky to do President Trump his favor of investigating the Bidens. Mr. Bolton, a Yale-trained lawyer, expressed grave concerns to Dr. Fiona Hill about the campaign being run by Mr. Giuliani. "Giuliani's a hand grenade who's going to blow everybody up."[91]

⭐ And in another boxing reference, House Intelligence Committee Chairman, Adam Schiff, was then asked whether or not he expects to address the White House's policy of non-cooperation with the investigation in the courts or just forge ahead with the investigation.

"In terms of how we will use litigation or not use litigation," Schiff answered, "we are not willing to allow the White House to engage us in a lengthy game of rope-a-dope in the courts, so we press forward." For those not familiar, the "rope-a-dope" is a boxing tactic famously used by Muhammad Ali in his 1974 fight against George Foreman, in which one fighter pretends to be stuck on the ropes in order to get his opponent to wear himself out with ineffective punches.[92] [and this might apply to witnesses who have yet to come forward to testify, namely, National Security Advisor John Bolton, White House acting Chief of Staff Mick Mulvaney and Secretary of State Mike Pompeo].[93]

✪ State Department on November 22, 2019, turns over hundreds of pages of documents that were not turned over to the investigative committee. These documents were turned over by court order under the Freedom of Information Act, and show a linkage between

Secretary of State Mike Pompeo, Rudolph Giuliani and Madaleine Westerhout, President Trump's assistant in the White House, of showing their involvement in the removal of the Ukranian ambassador, Marie Yovanovitch because of her resistance to their plan of pressuring the Ukranian president.[94] This paper trail confirms more specifically who was "in the loop" spoken of by Ambassador Sondland.

✪ Beyond the above, the turned-over documents reveal very little because they are largely redacted. These documents were requested through the Freedom of Information Act. The non-compliance by the executive office will most likely have to be appealed, creating a further stalling tactic.[95]

✪ While Mr. Trump claimed Yovanovitch refused to hang his portrait in the Ukrainian embassy, the *Washington Post* reported in September, 2017, federal buildings around the world, including U.S. embassies, were missing pictures of him and Pence because they hadn't yet decided when to sit for the photos. President Trump asked on *Fox News* why the

the House Republicans were being so kind to Ambassador Marie Yovanovitch?

He answered his own question when he stated "Well, sir, she's a woman. We have to be nice," the president claimed. "She's very tough."[96]

⭐ Is the President decrying this as a now, ranking member of the *#Push-Back Brigade* or as a form of Cancel Culture. "Cancel Culture became so central to the discourse in 2019 that even President Obama weighed in. The idea is that if you do something that others deem problematic, you automatically lose all your currency. Your voice is silenced. You're done."

Those who condemn 'Cancel Culture' usually imply that it's unfair and indiscriminate. Is President Trump decrying that because of the impeachment proceedings and alleged sexual affairs, his culture has been cancelled? "Since the *#MeToo* hashtag went viral in 2017, more women have spoken out about their experiences with sexual harassment and assault. While many people have applauded this movement, some men now say they fear even casual interactions with women will get them canceled."

⭐ "When political journalist Mark Halperin, who denied allegations of unwanted sexual contact but acknowledged that his "behavior was inappropriate and caused others pain," faced pushback over a new book, his publisher spoke to the *New York Post* decrying "this guilty-until-proven-innocent Cancel Culture where everyone is condemned to death or to a lifetime of unemployment based on an accusation that's 12 years old."[97]

⭐ The *#Push-Back Brigade* does not agree with President Trump's handling of the Yovanovitch scenario. She has always has been demonstrated by her peers to be an extremely competent foreign service officer.

⭐ Today, November 25, 2019, it was ruled on by U.S. District Court Judge Ketanji Brown Jackson that former White House counsel Donald McGahn, a key figure with first-hand knowledge of President Donald Trump's alleged efforts to short-circuit the Mueller investigation, must testify before Congress.[98]

✪ On 2/28 justices Griffith and Henderson ruled that McGhan need not testify in response to a Congressional subpoena[99] because to permit this would open a floodgate of litigation between branches rather than requiring the parties to "negotiate". But pertaining to McGahn and other White House officials who were subpoenaed, wasn't this what Congress attempted to do? These D.C. federal appeals court judges are Republican appointees. Dissenting judge Rogers was a democratic appointee. Here we find partisan politics entering an area of government, where they are supposed to be independent. This case can also be appealed to the Supreme Court of the United States just like the Trump tax return case and Deutsche Bank financial records cases.

The ruling equivocated over the Court's role in challenging Executive power. But a Supreme Court's reversal could once again affirm that role. It would uphold the subpoenas and open the door for testimony from some of the President's closest aides. These include former National Security Adviser John Bolton, and acting White House Chief of Staff Mick

Mulvaney. Mulvaney admitted the *quid-pro-quo* concerning Ukraine and said this kind of thing goes on all the time. "Get over it." John Bolton is in a win-win scenario. If he testifies and is shown to have knowledge that President Trump and Rudolph Giuliani initiated this idea of a trade-off, he would have been a hero of the impeachment proceedings and his book sales will soar. If he is kept from testifying by virtue of the acquittal in the impeachment trial without permission to testify, then his book sales will likewise soar. Ka-Ching, 'Mo Money'!! No complaints here with selling books and good old fashioned American capitalism.

Judge Ketanji Jackson had rejected the White House's claims of absolute immunity, saying the president "does not have the power" to prevent his aides from responding to congressional subpoenas.

"Today, this Court adds that this conclusion is inescapable precisely because compulsory appearance by dint of a subpoena is a legal construct, not a political one, and per the Constitution, no one is above the law," Jackson wrote in a lengthy ruling issued late Monday. The upshot of this is that the executive office and President Trump may be compelled to respond to Congressional subpoenas and testify. This is U. S. District Court Judge Jackson's decision. What is above it and which was decided on February 28 by the Washington, DC Court of Appeals is what has come later reversing her decision.

✪ House Democrats' new impeachment report revealed startling new details about one of President Trump's chief Republican defenders in Congress: Rep. Devin Nunes. The report portrayed how Nunes held repeated phone calls with key players at the center of the Ukraine scandal, including indicted Soviet-born businessman Lev Parnas and Trump's personal attorney Rudy Giuliani, at key moments of the Zalensky dialogue under investigation.[100]

✪ December 4, 2019, puts forth the riveting testimony at the beginning of the impeachment hearings. Professor Noah Feldman of Harvard University Law School in referencing acts of impeachment that may have been committed by President Trump says that one day in the afterlife we will be asked by the Founding Fathers, Madison, Hamilton,

Jay and the others how we decided and we would and should conclude that the President was guilty of impeachable offenses.[101]

★ The *#Push-Back Brigade* takes this moment to salute the words of House Speaker Nancy Pelosi, who, when asked the question if she hates President Trump (which is why the House voted for articles of impeachment) answered that she does not hate and "don't mess with me" in using the language of hate because she has never hated anyone. She says she has and feels compassion for President Trump but her job is to preserve and uphold the Constitution and our Democracy which is what she is doing. She is to be admired for taking and sticking to this position, on this issue. Amen to that.[102]

★ On Tuesday, December 10, 2019, the House of Representatives Judiciary Committee announced that they had approved two articles of impeachment against President Trump. He was charged with "...committing high crimes and misdemeanors," said Jerry Nadler, the chairman of the House Judiciary Committee. "The first article is for abuse of power. It is an impeachable offense for the president to exercise the powers of his public office to obtain an improper personal benefit while ignoring or injuring the national interest."

✪ I relate the following anecdote to my fellow Hot Tub Kingpins to emphasize a point of the failures in Constitutional government under President Trump. My student's name is Yasmine and she has a repugnance, as do many students today, to learning about the U.S. Constitution, the *Federalist Papers* and the Founding Fathers. The difficulty in building this kind of lesson plan is it goes to history that is 233 years old and, for students, not particularly relevant. The point that has to be taught and emphasized to students is that the Constitution was built as a living, breathing document flexible enough to accommodate the vicissitudes of time. Therein lies the dilemma for today's history teacher. It is imperative that today's history teacher get this right!!

Yasmine was waving her hands around in the air to describe the history she liked, i.e. WWI and WWII, and her response to whether she liked early American history was to describe it as "blech, no good!!" We certainly did hope that the House managers at the impeachment hearings could sway more of their Republican colleagues in the Senate to agree to allow for witnesses and evidence to be produced at the hearings. To allow the hearings to go forward without these proofs and witness testimony would set the Constitution on it's ear, dishonor the concepts of due process and cross-examination, and render the impeachment process void of any enforcement power under Article I (the legislative branch). This would allow Article II (the executive branch) to take precedence over all other articles in the Constitution including Article III (the judiciary branch).

✪ "When President Trump was caught as Congressman Nadler continues to read from the impeachment articles, when the House investigated and opened an impeachment inquiry, President Trump engaged in unprecedented, categorical, and indiscriminate defiance of the impeachment inquiry. This gives rise to the second article of impeachment, for obstruction of Congress. Here, too, we see a familiar pattern in President Trump's misconduct. A president who declares himself above accountability, above the American people, and above Congress's power of impeachment which is meant to protect against threats to our democratic institutions − is a president who sees himself as above the law. We must be clear: no one, not even the president, is above the law."[103]

★ Fittingly enough on Friday 13, the Supreme Court of the United States decided to take up the cases that President Trump has appealed from concerning production of his tax returns. They will hear arguments as to whether the executive office is immune from disclosing these records and decide the case in June. This gave him the delay to get the impeachment proceeings over and done with. ad SCOTUS refused to hear the case then the Circuit Court of Appeals decisions would have stood and he would have been forced to produce the records now. Those records will probably be redacted anyway if they are ever produced and the stall will continue into the next election cycle.[104]

✪ If President Trump had been forced to choose to enter his appearance now before Congress and push-back to demonstrate that the impeachment proceedings had not cancelled his culture of deniability, those of us in the Brotherhood and the Hot Tub Kingpins and the *#Push-Back Brigade* of the locker room would have more to relish arguing over it all in the name of collegiality. You can be sure of that!

✪ Shortly after midnight on January 3, President Trump, without consulting Congress, ordered drone strikes on Baghdad International Airport killing and martyring revered Iranian general Qassem Soleimani. The timing of the assassination seems highly suspicious with the impending impeachment trial set to commence.[105]

✪ John Bolton on January 6, 2020, alarmed with the pressure put on Ukraine, he said he would testify at the Senate impeachment trial if subpoenaed by Congress.[106]

✪ The House impeachment managers committed themselves to the "solemn and long" walk across the Capitol Rotunda to deliver the Articles of Impeachment to the Senate. Chief Justice of the Supreme Court John Roberts, presided and 99 Senators (1 absent) took their oaths to uphold the law while signing the book.[107]

✪ Lev Parnas gives a public interview to MSNBC's Rachel Maddow and reveals that he received his marching orders from No. 1, President Trump, to threaten the withholding of military aid to Ukraine unless President Zalensky announced an investigation into the Bidens.

Ultimately now the question remains: What would have happened if Parnas, Bolton, Mulvaney been permitted to testify at the impeachment hearing?[108]

Trump and Pompeo deny even knowing who Lev Parnas is despite many photo ops being taken among them for years.

✪ The General Administrative Office as an independent and non-biased party finds that the Trump Administration broke the law by witholding the Ukranian military aid.[109]

✪ Kenneth Starr and Alan Dershowitz were picked as defense lawyers at the impeachment trial. They both have their share of media notoriety which President Trump relishes. Starr prosecuted President Bill Clinton in his impeachment trial in 1998 and had more witnesses and documentary evidence that was provided to him. He now, as President Trump's defense lawyer, needs none to defend the case since President Trump has not turned any items over or allowed any administration officials to testify. Dershowitz was a member of the O.J. Simpson defense team. Both Starr and Dershowitz have had alleged sexual entanglements. Starr with the rape cases involving Baylor University football players during his tenure as president of the University. Dershowitz is alleged to have had his dalliances with the Jeffrey Epstein affair.[110, 111, 112]

✪ Starr had many witnesses available for the Clinton impeachment trial and much more extensive documentation keeping in mind the current White House staff's refusal to co-operate.

137

These lawyers would never be admitted to the *#Push-Back Brigade* because of their-seemingly 'unclean hands.'

⭐ Then again, you don't have to go back over 200 years. Professor John Mikhail, Georgetown University constitutional law professor, sees it as historically clear, contrary to what Dershowitz and the Trump defense team put forth "that lawmakers thought abuse of power was impeachable. Lawmakers during the impeachments of Presidents Andrew Johnson and Bill Clinton, and almost-impeachment of Richard Nixon thought so."

"All of these sources and others like them (e.g., Hamilton's remark on the 'abuse or violation of some public trust' in *Federalist Paper 65*) suggest that Dershowitz – and Trump – will have a hard time making a persuasive case that 'abuse of power' is not an impeachable offense," Mikhail wrote.[113]

⭐ Benjamin Wittes and Susan Hennessey in their new book, *Unmaking the Presidency* seem to be posing an apologist view toward the Trump Presidency which seem to analyze "Trump-era scandals and outrages in the deeper context of the presidency itself. How should we understand the oath of office when it is taken by a man who may not know what it means to preserve, protect, and defend something other than himself? What aspects of Trump are radically different from past presidents and what aspects have historical antecedents? When has he simply built on his predecessors' misdeeds, and when has he invented categories of misrule entirely his own?" These authors do not support a position that President Trump's ill-bekept knowledge of what defines a misdeed in office relieves him of his duties while in office. We, as human beings are held to moral precepts not the least of which just being the President of the United States.[114]

So as we steered into the headwinds of the storm called only the third impeachment trial of a president in our country's young history, we can only hope and pray that ultimately the ship is 'righted' and we begin the task of rebuilding our government for ourselves and in the eyes of the world.

So I say to all the Hot Tub Kingpins, *#MeToo*, *#Push-Back Brigade* and Wet Team members of the locker rooms across this great nation of our's, let us hope for the sake of our country that come election day, November, 2020, the American people collectively do the right thing.

The meeting of the Hot Tub Kingpins was called for Sunday after the White House defense outlined their opening statements. Ed, myself and Oscar took our respective spots in the hot tub and began the collegial arguments. We looked at the arguments of President Trump's team that he was not given due process and the right to cross-examine witnesses. Of course, I pointed out to them that the witnesses and documents were withheld from the proceedings by the order of President Trump. There was also fierce discussion over President Trump's claim that he did nothing wrong since he was seeking 'burden-sharing' over the military aid with our allies when he discussed Ukrainian corruption and the Bidens. I echoed the sentiments of Congressman Adam Schiff when I told my fellow kings that their Republican heroes might find t heir h ead o n a T rump pike[115] if they voted for witnesses, documentation and, worse yet, removal of President Trump from office.

I concluded with my hope that the Hot Tub Kingpins would continue to have the freedom to hold their meetings and voice their opinions freely and in a very democratic manner

"Mr. Trump's purported statement, as described by Bolton, would directly tie the US military aid freeze with the President's requests that Ukraine announce investigations into his political rivals – undermining a key pillar of the President's impeachment defense that the two circumstances are unrelated.[116]

In a series of late night tweets, President Trump denied claims he told Bolton aid to Ukraine was tied to an investigation of the Bidens. "I NEVER told John Bolton that the aid to Ukraine was tied to investigations into Democrats, including the Bidens. In fact, he never complained about this at the time of his very public termination," he tweeted.[117]

AFTERWORD

Where are all of these impeachment proceedings heading? Most people say nowhere and that the President will survive to run in 2020. That the best the Democrats can hope for is, like boxer Smokin' Joe Frazier said you gotta 'kill the body and the head will die,'[118] softening up the Democrats chances for 2020 presidential campaign. Only time will tell and maybe Mayor Bloomberg throwing his hat into the ring as a Democratic candidate. He filed to be a candidate on March 3, 2020, where 14 states primaries are on the table for Super Tuesday.[119] The question that I am raising is does our modern generation really care about what is happening to government and society in America.

Ronny Chieng, in his Netflix show, says all this fitness talk may be moot as well in the coming decades, that, in a way, fitness is on the way out with this new generation. "Never leave the house", Prime delivers anything to your house, same day delivery, drone or van, even if you want a single pencil delivered, it will come in 3 boxes. I want it NOW, not in 2 days or in 2 hours, NOW! You can put virtual reality headsets on, look at your iPad®, look at your smart phone, look at your smart watch, ALL AT THE SAME TIME!! No fitness training. We don't want to leave the house, just have artificial intelligence think of what you will want in the future and order it. It's a virtual world. NOW, maybe it is better to stay at home and socially distance yourself as a result of COVID-19. He says so much internet is making our culture stupid. Pregnant women in front of computer terminals, STUPID! Little babies using the internet, STUPID!

In your virtual world you ARE fit! In the future Chieng says, office buildings will have 'no computer' zones just like today we have 'no smoking areas'. Ronny Chieng is a very funny man but his prophesies could become a reality. Too much stupid information disbursed on today's Internet will make the viewing audience even more incapable of thinking for themselves. *GOOGLE, IT!!*

I have taught Civics and Colonial American History of the Founding Fathers for many years, my deep concern is whether this administration is excercising its Article II powers so broadly that the system of checks and balances built into our Constitution by the Founding

PRESIDENT TRUMP

Kingpin Pyramid System of Government

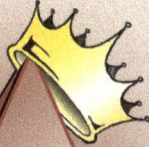

Executive
Order
Veto Power

Cultism
& Tribalism

Twitter
Social Media
Fake News

Belittling of Staff
Firing of Staff
Belittling Other Country Leaders

Misogyny
Stormy Daniels - *Access Hollywood*

Campaign Contributions
Misappropriation & withholding of aid

Kavanaugh • Gorsuch Appointees on the Supreme Court	McConnell & Graham in Senate	Pelosi in the House of Representatives

145

Fathers will be forever extinguished, with all power leading to the Presidency.

This proposed kingdom would undo centuries of democratic precedent and subject us as citizens to the whim of President Trump. I would point to Prince Harry and Meghan Markle in England as examples of how a mere 'wave of the royal hand' can remove one's established title.[120]

Call it the "Trump Triangle of Government" with President Trump controlling 90% of the triangle. The irony is that on November 19, the 156th Anniversary of President Lincoln's *Gettysburg Address* we recall Lincoln's words "Four score and seven years ago our fathers brought forth on this continent, a new nation, conceived in Liberty, and dedicated to the proposition that all men are created equal... that this nation, under God, shall have a new birth of freedom – and that government of the people, by the people, for the people, shall not perish from the earth..."[121]

In speaking to students, like Yasmine, they tell me they liked the part of the course where "every country was fighting" but found the Constitution and the founding fathers to be the 'real boring' part of U.S. History. This fear of our government perishing from the earth may portend what went on at the impeachment hearings among our Senators. I would have great difficulty constructing a lesson plan for students to assist them in learning what exactly is happening today with our sytem of government. A system with all power leading to the presidency. I certainly hope that we in America survive this crossroads in our government.

As the impreachment trial proceeded into the Whitehouse defense, I received a text from Big Ed one of the Hot Tub Kingpins and he decried, "what is going on with this impeachment?" My responsive text to him was, "Ed, leave me alone, go play racquetball and I'll meet you in the hot tub."

So, once ensconced in my spot in the hot tub, I grabbed one of the shower heads which are made by a company called 'Tuffman' (they even look like they were once used as microphones). The mikes looked like the Commando 450 showerheads in the Seinfeld episode. These showerheads were as big and powerful as the ones that Kramer, Jerry and Newman used (from the former Yugoslavia) but which were intended for showering down elephants.

I built my speech to its crescendo. And

said to all my fellow Hot Tub Kingpins "let's wait for the tax returns to be ruled on by the Supreme Court in the spring of 2020. It is Congress's oversight power under federal law and the Constitution as it relates to the I.R.S. and tax returns of the President that is being challenged here."

I am also quick to point out to the boys that President Trump's remarks about the deceased John Dingell, and "that he may be looking up from where he is now" after his wife voted for impeachment were highly inappropriate.[122]

Alexis de Tocqueville inscribed his vision of America in volume I, chapter 17 of his classic work on American political and social institutions, *Democracy in America*. Tocqueville, a French lawyer and member of the aristocracy, came to the United States in the spring of 1831. He traveled around Jacksonian America for nine months, and returned to France in the winter of 1832. The book continues to be one of the most far-reaching analyses of American culture ever written.

Tocqueville was convinced that the underlying reason for the success of democracy in America was the "manners" of the people. By manners, Tocqueville meant the value assumptions of the Americans, their overall "character of mind." He went on to say that manners referred to "the whole moral and intellectual condition of a people."[123] Clearly, today our government's manners are sorely lacking!! All of us, the Kingpins of the 70s standing alone and the current fitness and Locker Room Kings, are reacting to the acquittal of President Donald J. Trump at the impeachment trial. I hope for our sake, and certainly for our children's, that reason and balance can be restored to our government.

"If right doesn't matter, we're lost. If truth doesn't matter, we're lost. The framers couldn't protect us from ourselves if right and truth don't matter," Adam Schiff said. "And you know that what [Trump] did was not right."

He added: "No constitution can protect us if right doesn't matter anymore. And you know you can't trust this president to do what's right for this country. You can trust he will do what's right for Donald Trump. He'll do it now. He's done it before. He'll do it for the next several months. He'll do it in the election, if he's allowed to."

"And that," Schiff said, "is why Trump must be removed."

"**Right matters. And the truth matters**," Schiff said. "**Otherwise we are lost.**"

The speech caused Schiff's name to trend on Twitter, along with the phrases *#Right Matters* and *#TruthMatters*, His supporters praised the speech as one destined for the history books.[124]

As was previously recited in this book what followed the impeachment acquittal were the Bolton bombshell revelations from his book manuscript, *The Room Where It Happened*, which were leaked to the press. The excerpts revealed that he definitely overheard the *quid-pro-quo* -styled conversation between President Trump, Mick Mulvaney, acting Chief of Staff and Ukrainian President Zalensky." President Trump denies having ever had this conversation.

Bolton spokeswoman, Sarah Tinsley, said the draft of the book "was transmitted to the White House for pre-publication review by December 30, 2019, by the National Security Council."

Bolton's attorney Charles Cooper submitted this draft manuscript of the forthcoming book to the National Security Council. He said in a statement Sunday he submitted the manuscript on Bolton's behalf despite "our firm belief that the manuscript contained no information that could reasonably be considered classified."

Cooper also comes close to confirming the accuracy of the *Times* report, alleging that the "prepublication review process has been corrupted" and that "information has been disclosed by persons other than those properly involved in reviewing the manuscript."[125]

Hopefully, more pronouncements will be forthcoming.

Former White House Chief of Staff John Kelly attests to the sound character and integrity of John Bolton, and he knows him to always tell the unvarnished truth.[126] John Bolton, don't leave our republic because it needs you now more than ever. Call it the "Post-Impeachment Drama."

Ambassadors who were involved in the impeachment drama distance themselves from the chaos or are disgusted with its outcome.

✪ Ambassador William Taylor resigns his Ukraine posting.[127]

✪ Kurt D. Volker another integral part of the

impeachment probe previously resigned his post as the State Department's special envoy to Ukraine.[128]

✪ Marie Yovanovitch resigns her posting to the foreign service. She retires. Can't say that I blame her after the Trump instructions to Parnas and Giuliani were "Take her out."[129]

✪ It was revealed in a *New York Times* article, of January 31, that John Bolton says in his book that during a May 2019 Oval Office meeting, the president instructed him to call the president of Ukraine, Volodymyr Zelensky. The president wanted Bolton to make sure Zelensky would meet with his personal lawyer, Rudy Giuliani, who was planning a trip to Ukraine to talk to officials about investigations into the president's political opponents.

Bolton wrote that he never made that call. However, the timing of the meeting is significant because, according to Bolton, it took place more than two months prior to the now infamous July call Trump had with Zelensky and just a short time after Joe Biden entered the presidential race on April 25, 2019.

The other important revelation in the *Times'* reporting on the manuscript is Bolton's claim regarding who was at the May, 2019, Oval Office meeting: Giuliani, acting White House Chief of Staff Mick Mulvaney, White House Counsel Pat Cipollone, and Bolton were all in attendance. They all deny that such a meeting happened. The attorney, Cipollone, should never have argued the defense of the impeachment case having been in attendance at this meeting.[130]

- The Senate in a 51-49 vote decided there would be no witnesses or further documentation to be released.[131]

- At the State of Union speech, on February 5, 2020, President Trump refuses the extended offer from Nancy Pelosi to shake hands and at the conclusion of his speech, she rips up her copy of the speech.[132]

- At the vote on impeachment, Mitt Romney, a conservative Republican is the only Republican in the history of our country to vote for impeachment and removal of a sitting president of his own party. In a heart-felt speech, on February 5, 2020, he bespoke of the religious and moral beliefs that led him to that conclusion after analyzing the wrong-doing of President Trump.[133]

✪ In his East Room speech at the National Prayer Breakfast, on February 6, 2020, President Trump lashes out with vitriol against the Democrats which led them to the conclusion to vote for impeachment proceedings against him. He praises his great acquittal. He says he "does not like people who use prayer to justify their wrong doing" This is a direct shot across the bow at Mitt Romney and Nancy Pelosi.[134]

✪ February 7. Presidential Payback. Gordon Sondland is removed from post as ambassador to E.U., Lt. Col. Alexander Vindman removed from White House staff as a result of their testimony before the House Intelligence Committee[135]

The conversations of the Hot Tub Kingpins again imitate President Trump: "Hey, get out of this hot tub Colonel Vindman," I yelled at Oscar, "you're fired. – I only accept soldiers who fall on their swords, not their bone spurs in his heels for his 1-Y medical deferment (Trump), and die in battle, here on purple hearts (Vindman), and don't get captured by the enemy (John McCain), because that's not acceptable either!! And no more fruit-loops and cuckoo birds like that bald headed guy Sondland, he is not in my loop anymore! He wishes he had my hair!!"

A song for the Hot Tub Kingpins:

♫ *See You in November* ♫♪

I'll be alone each and every night.
While Pelosi, Schiff, Nadler and Schumer are
     in the House. I won't forget to tweet.

Bye-bye, so long, farewell, Vidman and Sondland.
Bye-bye, so long it's been fun for me now.
See you in November.
See you when the primaries are through.
Here we are (bye, baby, goodbye).
Saying goodbye from impeachment
     (bye, baby, goodbye).

Having a good time, but remember,
There is danger when my taxes come due.

I will see you in November.
Or lose you to summer loves named Mike, Joe,
    Bernie, Amy, Liz, Pete, Andrew, Hillary,
    or maybe even Mitt
(counting the days 'till we're on the stage)
(counting the hours and the minutes, too)

Bye, baby, goodbye (bye-bye, so long).
Have a good time but remember –
There is danger when my taxes come due.
I will see you in November.
Or lose you to summer loves named Mikey,
    Joey, Bernie, Amy, Lizzie or Petey, Andy,
    Hillary, or maybe even Mitt.

> Parody poem by the author;
> written by Sid Wayne and Sherman Edwards
> in 1959; most popularly recorded in 1966
> by The Happenings.

✪ All prosecutors in the Roger Stone case quit their positions because of the Department of Justice and Attorney General William Barr undercutting their sentencing recommendations on the heels of a President Trump tweet on February 11, 2020, which decried their proposals. The federal judge will have the absolute right to question why they have left the case and to set her own sentencing for Mr. Stone. "This situation has all the indicia of improper political interference in a criminal prosecution," Schumer said in a letter to Inspector General Michael Horowitz. "I therefore request that you immediately investigate this matter to determine how and why the Stone sentencing recommendations were countermanded, which Justice Department officials made this decision, and which White House officials were involved."

Ultimately President Trump has the power to pardon Stone which looms as a possibility for the future.[136]

⭐ February 13, 2020, Senator Elizabeth Warren and other leading Democrats are calling for the resignation of Attorney General William Barr or his impeachment for doing the bidding of President Trump in calling for a reduced sentence for Roger Stone, a close Trump ally.[137]

⭐ February 17, 2020, at Duke University, John Bolton states in an interview that he has been advised now to not comment on his book manuscript while it is being reviewed by the White House: The testimony he might have given at the impeachment trial may have tipped the scales in favor of impeachment.

Bolton, asked to comment on Trump's tweets about him, says "Nice try," and says he can't comment pending the White House review of his manuscript. He tweets, "but I can't talk about it. How fair is that?"[138]

⭐ Wednesday, February 19, Michael Bloomberg qualified for Democratic presidential debate in Las Vegas, paving the way for the former New York mayor's first appearance on stage with his 2020 rivals.

Bloomberg met the Democratic National Committee-mandated polling threshold on Tuesday with a *NPR/PBS NewsHour*/Marist survey finding the former New York mayor at 19% nationally.[139]

⭐ Today, in what many consider to be a far flung abuse of his executive powers, President Trump has pardoned Michael Milken, the junk bond defrauder of stock from 1990, and commuted the sentence of Rod R. Blagojevich, former governor of Illinois, who attempted to sell Barack Obama's vacated U.S.

Senatorial seat to the highest bidder and got caught doing it. Blagojevich did appear on President Trump's show, *The Apprentice* Trump says of him, "He served eight years in jail, a long time. He seems like a very nice person, don't know him."[140]

Ed, Oscar, and all of them are quick to point out that Blagojevich was great on the show which they all loved, and still has that great jet black hair style which they feel Trump really admires as they do.

✪ We know that while he was governor, he never had a bad hair day, sometimes taking a full day to coiff and tint his hair jet black, which is now completely grey.[141]
Milken is bald as is Bernard Kerik, former NYC Police Commisioner who also had his tax fraud conviction and sentence commuted.

✪ The Hot Tub Kingpins were exulting in the outcome of the Democratic Party debate on February 19, 2020. They howled over the exchange when Senator Amy Klubuchar couldn't remember the name of the Mexican President when questioned by Mayor

Pete Buttigieg and she turned to him and said, "Are you – calling me dumb, Pete? Are you mocking me? – And you're so perfect, you remember everything?"[142]

★ Is former N.Y.C. Mayor Mike Bloomberg out of the presidential race before he is even in?? The seniors of the Hot Tub Kingpins think so. "Those 2 stents you had, Bernie, mine were 35 years ago" retorted Bloomberg. They think that President Trump is loving the result of the Nevada debate and is now in position to win his second term. I envision him seeking a third term and beyond. He will seek a change to the Twenty-second Amendment to allow him to run for an unlimited number of terms in office. Oh boy, what a thought that is!! The fracking of natural gas and oil, coal burning, and mining will continue to despoil our environment.[143]

Bloomberg takes heavy blows from other candidates on the debate stage, and the question is: can he get off the canvas to fight again. He would not disclose the nature and number of N.D.A.'s he has entered into with female employees, "They signed those agreements and we will live with it." Senator Warren accused him of calling women "horse-faced lesbians and fat broads." The *#Me-Too Movement* was again turned on its ear during this debate. His tax returns are still forthcoming as he makes a haughty reference to not being able to use Turbo Tax to do them.[144]

Were these K.O. blows from candidate, Elizabeth Warren, the metaphorical equivalency of Roberto Durán's fearsome tenacity and powerful punches that earned him the nickname "Manos de Piedra" (Hands of Stone)? They finished off Mayor Bloomberg for sure, and possibly Joe Biden as candidates.[145]

Or is it shaping up that Joe Biden is gonna be the Danny "Little Red" Lopez, coming back to knock out his opponents. The Comeback Kid, as it were, of this primary season, coming off the mat to knock out his opponents! I tell all my colleagues in the hot tub that I had occasion to speak with Danny and he told me that he kept on fighting even when knocked down till his legs gave out on him in the Salvador Sanchez championship fights where he, himself, was knocked out twice. I do hope that one of these Democratic candidates similarly come off the stage in these primaries to win the nomination outright and fight for preservation of the presidency.

If not in the future, the Democrats will have to rely on a candidate like present governor of California, Gavin Newsom. I have seen him first hand connect with college graduates by reponding to their email suggestions for change. The only problem with Newsom is that he has so many problems to deal within California that he needs to first get that house in order before turning to the national stage. I want to see how he handles the California budget, the environmental issues, the issue of high speed mass transit and immigration and sanctuary cities among many others. So my hot tub mates stay tuned.

✪ The Roger Stone sentencing was heard on February 20. Judge Amy Berman Jackson says sarcastically that it is usually the defense that argues to a reduction of the sentencing guidelines not the attorney general's office. Her ruling on the issue of sentencing conforms to those recommended by the prosecutors in the case, but reduces the sentencing somewhat taking into consideration the defendant's age. Her sentence is forty months, two years probation and fines. The sentence validates the Muller investigation, Stone's lying to Congress and manipulating witnesses as the judge says "The truth still matters." Again, a Stone pardon would seem likely to be part of the "watergate" of pardons which have been issued by President Trump this week.[146]

⭐ *The New York Times* has reported that just as Robert Mueller made findings about the 2016 election, it is now found that the Russians have been complicit, again, in hacking the United States election process for 2020. President Trump has attempted to prevent disclosure to Congress and, in particular Congressman Adam Schiff who led the impeachment trial as head of the intel committee and who President Trump feels will "weaponize" this information against him. In the February 13 briefing, Shelby Pierson, point person in charge of the investigation, reported her findings of Russia's hacking activities. President Trump was angry about the disclosures and has removed his national intellgence chief, Joseph Maguire, and appointed Richard Grenell as the temporary director of national intelligence.

Grinnell has no intelligence experience whatsoever having previously been ambassador to Germany.[147]

I do hope that no pardons will be forthcoming by President Trump to Julian Assange and Wikileaks for, as a condition for Assange stating publicly, that there was no hacking in our 2016 elections and the Democratic National Committee in favor of Donald Trump.[148]

✪ The Julian Assange Wikileak connection about the Russian hacking of the Democratic National Committee was also the subject of the Roger Stone case. Stone was connected to Assange and/or Wikileaks itself on the Russian hacking in the 2016 election.[149]

In the 1993 movie, *Schindler's List*, the following pardoning dialogue is emblematic for President Trump's spree of pardoning in the week of February 20, 2020, and I thought of it while having one of my lucid morning swims with the Wet Team:

Oskar Schindler: Power is when we have every justification to kill, and we don't.

Amon Goeth: You think that's power?

Oskar Schindler: That's what the Emperor said. A man steals something, he's brought in before the Emperor, he throws himself down on the ground. He begs for his life, he knows he's going to die. And the Emperor... pardons him. This worthless man, he lets him go.

Amon Goeth: I think you are drunk.

Oskar Schindler: That's power, Amon. That is power.

Then Goeth, the German Kommandant with a penchant for killing innocents, proceeds to pardon everyone. He pardons his stable boy who mishandles his horse saddle. He pardons Lisiek, the house boy, who failed to clean his bathtub. And, after pardoning Lisiek, he changes his mind and shoots him anyway as he walks away...

Convention Forecasts for Milwaukee, 2020

THE DEMOCRATIC CONVENTION IN MILWAUKEE THIS SUMMER

1. Hillary Clinton gets written in by ballot and nominated for the Presidency by the Democrats. She defeats Donald Trump in his re-election bid.

2. Joe Biden and either Amy Klobuchar or Kamala Harris as the Democratic ticket, join forces to take on and defeat Donald Trump for the Presidency

3. John Bolton continues to talk about his involvement in the White House and it turns out that he, in fact, is the Whistle-Blower.

4. Governor Cuomo of New York has done such a splendid job of dealing with the virus epicenter in his state that many are projecting his becoming a write-in candidate after the first balloting at a brokered convention. I just listened to Governor Andrew Cuomo of New York again reiterate absurdidly of how the 50 states and the federal government are bidding against each other for the ventilator supplies which will help sustain the fight against the spread of the corona-virus. He makes note of the fact that his brother, CNN news commentator Chris Cuomo has now tested positive for COVID-19

5. Pat A. Cippolone is brought up on disbarment proceedings for having been in attendance at the meeting in May, 2019, over the Ukraine affair. That meeting was attended by all the guys. He then appears to have had a conflict of interest when he undertook the defense of President Trump at the impeachment trial over what John Bolton, national security adviser, President Trump, Mick Mulvaney, acting White House Chief of Staff, Rudolph Giuliani, President Trump's personal lawyer, discussed in the May 2019 meeting over the Ukraine affair.[150]

6. After the chaos of the pandemic and the collapse of the economy, President Trump decides not to run in 2020 because of the corona virus. He is heard to utter the word "No más, no más" echoing those artful words of

Roberto Durán who chose not to get out of his corner in the second Sugar Ray Leonard fight, Superdome, Houston, November 1980.[151]

7. In the alternative, as Joe Biden warns, President Trump may attempt to kickback the election since his poll numbers have dropped so seriously because of the pandemic and economy. This would be constitutionally illegal to do without an amendment to the Constitution. [152]

Recent Vintage Trumpisms

On the onset of the coronavirus pandemic, President Trump tells us to bail out, and not touch handrails, and wash our hands a lot to counter the coronavirus. He says we have it now under control. This despite the fact that the CDC says, as yet, it is unknown how much it will spread among the 'community.' Without the proper amount of test kits and face masks for the virus they cannot get a handle of the virus's impact here in the United States.[153]

Bear in mind, however, that the President wants no restrictors on our showers, so they don't drip, drip, drip on his 'beautiful head of hair.' **Geez!!**[154]

And so it came to pass that the Hot Tub Kingpins came together for one last time on March 1, 2020, and had a discussion about the disastrous stockmarket dip of 4,500 points in the past week. Oscar, who we also now call 'blip' man because he says the stock market crash and global warming are mere 'historical blips.'

I interjected to all the Hot Tub Kingpins that it must be a mere coincidence that these events are happening now at this precise time in history.

At this March 1, 2020 meeting the discussion ensued about the horrendous stock market plunge in the past week. The 'blip' says don't be a 'putz' invest now in some option 'puts'. He is a very negative guy cause you are betting the market and a particular stock will go down to a certain value by a certain date. It is negative to bet the market to go down. Not a good forecast for our economy!

I also mentioned again to the boys, as I had done previously on numerous occasions, that global warming was not also just the result of an 'historical blip'; the fracking, coal mining and burning, oil refining and continued use of plastics were major contributors to global warming.

If you put Vice-President Mike Pence in charge of scientific protocol and a national health plan, you are making a colossal mistake. He believes that religion can explain the virus and global warming. Not science!

Beyond the mishandling of the coronavirus and the appointment of the Vice-President to head the health program, President Trump is seeking to score political points by wearing his hat and windbreaker to attend the CDC press conference. Despite the fact that our country does not have enough testing kits to attend all the sick, President Trump wears his windbreaker and red 'Make America Great Again' hat. This is his emergency crisis outfit which he used in the hurricane in Puerto Rico and he pulls it out of the drawer for each of his crisis situations. What's that about? He was actually indoors at the time of this news conference!

He is also mishandling the outbreak by not giving care to the passengers onboard the cruise ship. President Trump wants to keep the ship off the coast of California from docking. Since 21 of the 46 passengers tested on the

Princess Diamond are positive for the coronavirus, he wants to keep his numbers down for political purposes. He admits wanting to keep the numbers down this way.[155] Unfortunately for us he's playing the numbers game a political numbers game with peoples' lives.

Now for further updated news and a positive spin to the election year, Vice-President Joe Biden won 9 primaries on Super Tuesday, March 3, 2020, and his delegate lead over Bernie Sanders now stands at 453 to 373. He has surged toward the nominating convention in Milwaukee. His big victories also confirm the prognostications of the Trump team in that-their attacks made against him and his son, Hunter, over the Ukrainian affair have failed.[156]

At 10:11 ET, Mike Bloomberg quits the race. On April 8, 2020 Bernie Sanders quits the Democratic race for President.[157,158]

The Hot Tub Kingpins stay friends but sometimes I feel like I am living in an alternate universe. Winston Smith in '1984' can you hear me? The locker room and club are now officially closed because of the Pandemic.

I hope for our sake, and certainly for our children's, that reason and balance can be restored to our government.

There is a national emergency spreading the COVID-19 virus. President Trump finally realizes that the virus could not be stopped without massive testing and social distancing. So during the "Silence of the Pandemic," I socially distance myself and read *Dark Towers*, written by David Enrich.[159]

I do not usually read other books while I am endeavoring to complete my own. However, this book intrigued me because it is an historical analysis of Deutsche Bank, a Frankfurt, Germany institution.

Deutsche Bank was involved in financing the Holocaust and building Auschwitz. It chronicles the suicide hangings of a number of its upper level executives because of toxic loans. I think about this city where my mother and family grew up prizing a tomato as a gift in the Great Depression while this bank plundered the world of finance.

Most importantly, it portrays the linkage today between the bank and the Trump family. Donald Trump could not obtain loans because he had defaulted on so many and filed for bankruptcy four times. While one division of the Bank was suing him for default on loans and personal guarantees, another division was loaning more money to him, his sons and Jared Kushner to build golf courses and hotels in Florida, Chicago and Washington, DC.

What comes under investigation now is the nature of these loans. Was the underlying paper sold to Russian banks, oligarchs and the money laundered in these mirror trades, going into the loan as roubles and through Cyprus and then transforming them to dollars in the United States? Was the President under the control of the Russian oligarchs and banks at the time of his election victory in 2016?

As I mentioned earlier in this book, the District Attorney of New York has subpoenaed the Trump tax returns for the past years. His refusal to comply is now the subject of the case which is before the United States Supreme Court. It will be argued at some point this Spring and decided, hopefully, before the November election.[160] I have not seen the Hot Tub Kingpins since the national emergency began but I am looking forward to countless hours of discussion once the virus is contained.

Now more than ever we are explicitly told to 'socially distance' ourselves from our fellow man. I guess if the streets of major cities are empty, and health clubs, gyms, churches, non-essential businesses like professional athletics and theater have shuttered their doors, the distance becomes an irrelevancy. This pandemic has not yet reached its zenith at the time of this book's printing.

The coffee which was tested on the battlefields between the Union and Confederacy and, later, in global theaters of war will not bring us relief because government will not allow us to congregate anymore in Starbucks® or Dunkin Donuts.® We are prohibited from clustering at all for health concerns and we may find ourselves penalized if we choose to remain in groups.

Basketball rims are being taken down in our cities and playgrounds are being taped up for security purposes. This is the modern day version of the wars which created divisions among us in past history. Field hospitals are now springing up all around us: the Javits Center, the West Lawn Tennis Club, Central Park in New York City are all being outfitted as health facilities. One can only speculate and hope that this scourge will soon run its course.

We are now relegated, once again, to the

historical battle of states' rights vs. federal rights, as the states battle among themselves and with the federal agencies for protective health gear to treat those who have fallen ill.

Battlefields, trenches, culture-clashes, gender clashes and partisan politics pale in comparison to this invisible enemy which is returning us to the caveman paradigm from whence this book began. Try to manage your risk factors as best you can. Get rid of your Fettleibigkeit!

\

THE END

STAY, SAFE, SANE AND, ABOVE ALL ELSE,

KEEP FIT

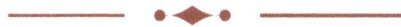

END NOTES

1 *https://www.merriam-webster.com/dictionary/obese*

2 *https://en.wikipedia.org/wiki/Vitali Klitschko*

3 *https://www.artofmanliness.com/articles/the-history-of-physical-fitness/*

4 *https://en.wikipedia.org/wiki/Otzi*

5 *National Geographic* article in September, 2019, edition on The Arctic

6 *https://qz.com/1366826/parts-of-the-arctic-that-used-to-never-thaw-are-now-melting/*

7 *ESPN-The Magazine*, October, 2019

8 *https://www.youtube.com/watch?v=9DxlAuKP_FI*

9 *https://www.artofmanliness.com/articles/the-history-of-physical-fitness/*

10 ibid -9

11 *https://humwp.ucsc.edu/cwh/brooks/coffee-site/1400-1800.html*

12 *https://www.bostonglobe.com/lifestyle/2014/09/11/presidential-history-coffee/Wv2SfehMBGi8uyAGcMP6tN/story.html*

13   *https://www.wnd.com/2017/03/the-stupendous-logistical-feat-of-henry-knox/*

14   *https://thereformedbroker.com/2011/07/04/a-message-from-henry-knox/*

15   *hudsonrivervalley.wordpress.com/2015/03/23/re-remembering-the-henry-knox-trail*

16   *http://www.newenglandhistoricalsociety.com/love-letters-lucy-henry-knox/*

17   *https://knoxtrailcoffee.com/pages/about-us*

18   *https://jeffersonbackroads.com/2014/03/a-brief-history-of-fort-jones/*

19   *https://www.battlefields.org/learn/articles/coffee-and-civil-war-soldier*

20   *https://civilwartalk.com/threads/william-mckinley-coffee-and-antietam.21918/*

21   *https://www.theguardian.com/film/2020/feb/22/clint-eastwood-bloomberg-president-trump*

22   *https://truewestmagazine.com/cowboy-coffee/*

23   *https://en.wikipedia.org/wiki/Eight_O%27Clock_Coffee*

24   *https://www.npr.org/sections/thesalt/2017/04/06/522071853/in-wwi-trenches-instant-coffee-gave-troops-a-much-needed-boost*

25 ibid. - 24

26 *https://www.elliscoffee.com/*

27 op. cit. - 24

28 op. cit. - 24

29 *https://www.ideastream.org/news/in-wwi-trenches-instant-coffee-gave-troops-a-much-needed-boost*

30 *https://www.kpbs.org/news/2017/apr/06/in-wwi-trenches-instant-coffee-gave-troops-a-much/*

31 *https://taskandpurpose.com/history/coffee-important-army-gi-joe-gave-name*

32 *op.cit -30*

33 *https://bleacherreport.com/articles/761050-detroit-pistons-the-five-baddest-boys-of-the-bad-boys-era#slide5*

34 *https://vault.si.com/vault/1991/11/18/dangerous-games-in-the-age-of-aids-many-pro-athletes-are-sexually-promiscuous-despite-the-increasing-peril*

35 *https://www.cnn.com/2019/11/10/business/goldman-sachs-apple-card-discrimination/index.html*

36 *https://www.miamiherald.com/news/politics-government/state-politics/article189152134.html*

37 *https://www.dailywire.com/news/watch-woke-artists-rewrite-responsible-lyrics-baby-amanda-prestigiacomo*

38   https://www.npr.org/2020/02/24/805258433/harvey-weinstein-found-guilty-of-rape-but-acquitted-of-most-sexual-assault-charg

39   https://www.newsweek.com/metoo-movement-gender-backlash-men-maintain-hierarchies-power-1449740

40   ibid - 3

41   https://www.cnn.com/2019/11/17/politics/michael-bloomberg-stop-and-frisk-apology/index.html

42   https://en.wikipedia.org/wiki/Dot-com_bubble

43   https://phys.org/news/2016-06-dyprosiumif-goodbye-smartphones-mri-scans.html

44   https://www.history.com/news/the-myth-of-ponce-de-leon-and-the-fountain-of-youth

45   https://www.cbsnews.com/news/harvard-geneticist-george-church-goal-to-protect-humans-from-viruses-genetic-diseases-and-aging-60-minutes-2019-12-08/

46   https://www.cbsnews.com/news/harvard-scientist-george-church-talks-about-accepting-donations-from-jeffrey-epstein-60-minutes-2019-12-08/

47   https://www.nationsonline.org/oneworld/chinese_customs/TsaiShen.htm

48   https://www.theguardian.com/science/2011/jul/26/cryonics-pioneer-robert-ettinger-dies

49   https://www.youtube.com/watch?v=AF-KhUkT_kc

50 *https://abcnews.go.com/GMA/story?id=1248088&page=1*

51 *https://sabr.org/gamesproj/game/june-9-1946-ted-williams-hits-502-foot-red-seat-home-run-fenway-park*

52 *https://www.scienceabc.com/humans/movies/captain-america-survive-frozen-ice-70-years-suspended-animation-cryonics.html*

53 *https://en.wikipedia.org/wiki/Suspended_animation_in_fiction#Literature*

54 *https://superheroesmodernmyths.wordpress.com/2015/02/08/captain-americas-role-within-american-wartime-patriotism-and-propaganda/*

55 *https://time.com/5720772/running-helps-you-live-longer/*

56 *https://business.fit/brief-history-of-fitness/*

57 *https://en.wikipedia.org/wiki/Joe_Morrison*

58 *https://en.wikipedia.org/wiki/Marty_Glickman#Early_life_and_education*   There were many others that I admired greatly.

59 *https://en.wikipedia.org/wiki/Yang_Chuan-kwang*

60 *http://www.jeremylin.net/*

61 *https://en.wikipedia.org/wiki/Michael_Chang*

62 *https://en.wikipedia.org/wiki/Michelle_Kwan*

63 *nypost.com/2019/09/16/trumps-tax-returns-subpoenaed-by-manhattan-das-office-source-says/*

64 *https://www.npr.org/2019/09/25/764390138/the-latest-on-the-trump-ukraine-controversy*

65 *https://www.cnn.com/2019/10/17/politics/mick-mulvaney-quid-pro-quo-donald-trump-ukraine-aid/index.html*

66 *https://www.thedailybeast.com/gordon-sondland-told-house-trump-offered-a-quid-pro-quo-to-ukraine-wsj*

67 *https://www.aol.com/article/news/2019/11/08/trump-on-dems-impeachment-probe-were-kicking-their-ass/23856463/*

68 *https://www.youtube.com/watch?v=JE7ZL5H8IDw*

69 *https://en.m.wikipedia.org/wiki/Hanged,_drawn_and_quartered*

70 *https://www.npr.org/2019/11/13/778824788/read-william-taylors-opening-statement-in-public-impeachment-hearing*

71 *ttps://www.foxnews.com/media/trump-reportedly-traveling-to-new-york-for-mma-fight-on-saturday*

72 *https://www.usatoday.com/story/news/politics/2019/11/01/why-president-donald-trump-moving-new-york-florida/4120843002/*

73 *https://www.legendsofamerica.com/we-slang/13/*

74   *National Geographic* article in September, 2019, edition on The Arctic.

75   *https://qz.com/1366826/parts-of-the-arctic-that-used-to-never-thaw-are-now-melting/*

76   *https://www.theguardian.com/us-news/2019/nov/04/donald-trump-tax-returns-appeals-court*

77   *https://www.reuters.com/article/us-usa-trump-banks/court-directs-banks-to-provide-trump-financial-records-to-house-democrats-idUSKBN1Y71V0*

78   *https://thehill.com/regulation/court-battles/467108-trump-attorney-president-could-shoot-someone-on-fifth-avenue-and-not*

79   *https://www.usatoday.com/story/news/politics/2019/11/01/why-president-donald-trump-moving-new-york-florida/4120843002/*

80   *https://www.nationalreview.com/news/trumps-threat-to-cut-california-wildfire-aid-sparks-bipartisan-alarm/*

81   *https://hillreporter.com/report-drug-smugglers-are-cutting-through-new-sections-of-trumps-border-wall-50043*

82   *https://bbc.in/2UEXYb1*

83   *https://www.motherjones.com/politics/2019/11/roger-stone-was-just-convicted-on-all-counts/*

84　*https://en.wikipedia.org/wiki/Festivus*

85　*https://www.businessinsider.com/gordon-sondland-trump-ukraine-investigation-state-department-aide-david-holmes-2019-11*

86　*https://cbs4indy.com/2019/11/17/trump-visit-to-walter-reed-not-protocol-for-routine-visit-source-says/*

87　*https://www.redstate.com/bradslager/2019/11/19/734891/*

88　*https://slate.com/news-and-politics/2019/11/gordon-sondland-testimony-impeachment-hearing-pompeo-giuliani-september.html*

89　*https://www.usatoday.com/story/news/politics/2019/11/20/sondland-pence-pompeo-trump-plan-pressure-ukraine-emails/4248107002/*

90　*https://www.bbc.com/news/av/world-us-canada-50494391/trump-impeachment-inquiry-president-re-enacts-sondland-call*

91　*https://www.politicususa.com/2019/10/15/john-bolton-guiliani-ukraine.html*

92　*https://en.wikipedia.org/wiki/Rope-a-dope*

93　*https://www.conservativereview.com/news/schiff-exec-branch-staffers-defy-impeachment-subpoenas-build-powerful-case-trump-obstruction/*

94 *https://www.americanoversight.org/state-department-releases-ukraine-documents-to-american-oversight*

95 *https://publicintegrity.org/national-security/ukraine-documents-dod-omb-foia/*

96 *https://www.cbsnews.com/news/trump-claims-marie-yovanovitch-refused-to-hang-portrait-in-embassy-in-ukraine/*

97 *https://time.com/5735403/cancel-culture-is-not-real/*

98 *https://www.usatoday.com/story/news/politics/2019/11/25/judge-former-white-house-counsel-don-mcgahn-must-testify-before-congress/4295727002/*

99 *https://www.usatoday.com/story/news/politics/2020/02/28/ex-trump-counsel-don-mcgahn-doesnt-have-testify-court-rules/4678695002/*

100 *https://www.vice.com/en_us/article/wjwv9z/dems-impeachment-report-puts-devin-nunes-in-middle-of-trumps-ukraine-scandal*

101 *https://www.bloomberg.com/opinion/articles/2019-12-07/what-the-founding-fathers-thought-about-impeachment*

102 *https://www.youtube.com/watch?v=nO9syIIJhyE*

103 *https://www.cnbc.com/2019/12/10/house-democrats-announce-articles-of-impeachment-against-trump.html*

104   https://www.nbcnews.com/politics/politics-news/
supreme-court-agrees-hear-trump-appeals-
subpoena-fights-over-financial-n1101901

105   https://nypost.com/2020/01/02/trump-ordered-
strike-that-killed-iranian-gen-qassim-soleimani-
pentagon/

106   https://www.cbsnews.com/news/john-bolton-trump-
impeachment-trial-former-adviser-says-today-hell-
testify-if-subpoenaed-by-senate-2020-1-6/

107   https://www.npr.org/2020/01/15/796240568/house-
set-to-vote-to-send-trump-impeachment-articles-to-
senate

108   www.politico.com/news/2020/01/16/lev-parnas-
trump-impeachment-trial-099781

109   https://jonathanturley.org/2020/01/16/gao-declares-
trumps-action-on-ukraine-aid-to-be-unlawful/
comment-page-1/

110   https://www.usnews.com/news/politics/
articles/2020-01-17/trump-taps-kenneth-starr-alan-
dershowitz-for-impeachment-defense-team

111   https://www.espn.com/college-football/story/_/
id/17345898/ken-starr-resigns-law-professor-severs-
ties-baylor-bears

112   https://www.newsweek.com/alan-dershowitz-
jeffreyepstein-perfect-sex-life-rape-1450140

113   https://abcnews.go.com/Politics/video/trump-team-presents-impeachment-trial-68587998

114   https://www.brookings.edu/events/unmaking-the-presidency/

115   https://abcnews.go.com/Politics/democratschiffs-head-pike-comment-draws-outrage-gop/story?id=68527054

116   https://www.politico.com/news/2020/01/27/trump-john-bolton-ukraine-aid-105942

117   https://www.politico.com/news/2020/01/26/bolton-ukraine-aid-impeachment-witnesses-105658

118   http://thinkexist.com/quotation/kill_the_body_and_the_head_will_die/346821.html

119   https://www.desmoinesregister.com/story/news/elections/presidential/caucus/2019/11/08/michael-bloomberg-presidential-race-alabama-democratic-primary-iowa-caucuses-2020/2534688001/

120   https://www.iheart.com/content/2020-01-21-the-queen-almost-stripped-harry-and-meghan-of-duke-duchess-titles-too/

121   https://www.historynet.com/gettysburg-address-text

122   https://www.nydailynews.com/news/national/nydonald-trump-john-dingle-debbie-dingle-20191219- mt3shhilrrfdlf

123   *https://theimaginativeconservative.org/2016/07/ what-would-tocqueville-think-of-trump.html*

124   *https://www.365news.com/2020/01/masterful- twitter-users-hail-adam-schiffs-powerful-case-for- trumps-removal/*

125   *https://www.msn.com/en-us/news/politics/new-york- times-bolton-book-draft-says-trump-tied-ukraine- aid-to-political-investigations/ar-BBZlXAR*

126   *https://thehill.com/homenews/administration/ 483043-john-bolton-defends-john-kelly-after- trump-criticism*

127   *https://politicaldig.com/ambassador-bill- taylorresigns-from-top-post-in-ukraine-after- testifyingagainst-trump/*

128   *https://www.rt.com/news/469796- ukraineambassador-resigns-impeachement/*

129   *https://www.cnn.com/2020/01/31/politics/marie- yovanovitch-retires/index.html*

130   *https://thehill.com/homenews/senate/480909-trump- denies-asking-bolton-to-put-zelensky-and-giuliani-in- contact*

131   *https://variety.com/2020/politics/news/ senateimpeachment-trump-vote-acquitall- 1203488838/*

132 *https://www.usatoday.com/story/news/politics/ 2020/02/04/state-union-president-trumpwont-shake-nancy-pelosis-hand/4660937002/*

133 *https://www.cnbc.com/2020/02/06/trump-lashes-out-during-national-prayer-breakfast-speech-after-acquittal.html*

134 *https://www.usatoday.com/story/news/politics/2020/ 02/06/trump-uses-national-prayer-breakfastblast-impeachment-supporters/4676811002/* 125 NBC news.com

135 *https://www.justsecurity.org/68586/the-early-edition-february-10-2020/*

136 *https://www.politico.com/news/magazine/2020/02/ 27/trump-pardon-roger-stone-constitution-117757*

137 *https://thehill.com/homenews/senate/482764-warren-renews-call-for-barr-to-resign*

138 *https://www.cnn.com/2020/02/17/politics/john-bolton-white-house-book/index.html*

139 *https://www.wrcbtv.com/story/41714167/bloomberg-qualifies-for-wednesdays-democratic-debate-his-first*

140 *https://www.wsj.com/articles/trump-has-commuted-sentence-of-rod-blagojevich-11582051259*

141 *https://www.dailymail.co.uk/news/article-3032626/ He-s-not-dye-ing-prison-Shamed-Illinois-politician-Rod-Blagojevich-pictured-snow-white-hair-serves-time.html*

142 https://thehill.com/homenews/campaign/483781-klobuchar-shuts-down-buttigieg-criticism-are-youcalling-me-dumb

143 https://www.usatoday.com/story/news/politics/elections/2020/02/27/mike-bloomberg-calls-bernie-sanders-do-same/4893947002/

144 https://dailycaller.com/2020/02/19/fat-broads-lesbians-warren-bloomberg-trump/

145 https://www.biography.com/athlete/roberto-duran

146 https://www.nbcnews.com/politics/justicedepartment/trump-associate-roger-stone-sentenced3-years-4-months-prison-n1138516

147 https://wgno.com/news/russia-is-looking-to-help-trump-win-in-2020-security-official-tells-lawmakers/

148 https://www.theguardian.com/media/2020/feb/19/donald-trump-offered-julian-assange-pardon-russia-hack-wikileaks

149 https://www.independent.co.uk/news/world/americas/us-politics/roger-stone-donald-trump-julian-assange-russia-wikileaks-us-election-2016-a8254636.html

150 https://lawandcrime.com/impeachment/cipollone-must-come-clean-calls-for-disciplinary-action-against-wh-counsel-intensify/

151 *https://en.wikipedia.org/wiki/Roberto_
Dur%C3%A1n_vs._Sugar_Ray_Leonard_II*

152 *https://www.politico.com/news/2020/04/23/biden-
trump-2020-delay-coronavirus-206142*

153 *https://abcnews.go.com/Politics/trump-coronavirus-
control-us-problem/story?id=
69198905story?id=69198905*

154 *https://www.yahoo.com/entertainment/trump-
beautiful-head-hair-complaints-202645888.html*

155 *https://www.businessinsider.com/trump-keep-
passengers-on-grand-princess-cruise-ship-
coronavirus-2020-3*

156 *https://www.youtube.com/watch?v=5CAw1d9vuns*

157 *https://video.search.yahoo.com/yhs/search?fr=yhs-
iba-syn&hsimp=yhs-syn&hspart=iba&p=Mike+Bl
umberg+resigns+from+the+race#id=1&vid=e43f74
904987e042e0ee0192484c9737&action=click*

158 *https://www.nbcnews.com/politics/2020-
election/bernie-sanders-drops-out-presidential-
race-n1155156*

159 *https://www.salon.com/2020/03/14/financial-
reporter-examines-deutche-banks-disturbing-
relationship-with-donald-trump_partner/*

160 *https://finance.yahoo.com/news/coronavirus-delays-
us-supreme-court-154704599.html*

Endorsement

for

Locker Tales

Thanks for passing this along, I enjoyed the manuscript.

It's an entertaining and educational trip down our collective "historical memory lane" and reflects the simplicity of social interaction (in reference to coffee) and the transcendence into the superficial societal norms of today.

When there was ACTUAL conflict (war, famine, death), the focus on coffee was an interesting observation as a subtle keystone of progress.

Today, "1st-world problems" reflect how devoid true conflict in our culture actually is. I enjoyed the read!

Dash Kellner
Founder of Swolenormous

Endorsements

for the

Soccer Tales Trilogy

Just as with *Locker Tales*, Mr. Freimark's *The Soccer Tales Trilogy*, has also taken the reader on travels through a timeline of history. We learned that the sport of soccer originated in ancient China and later was adapted to life in the New World and Meso-America.

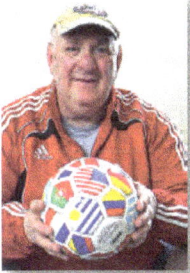

America is struggling to emerge with its own national personae of the game. In providing his stewardship to the youth programs the Shoelace Monster has fashioned it into one of the fastest growing sports of our country. Local stars like Carli Lloyd and Christian Polisic and successful coaches such as Anthony DiCicco add to its luster. See some of the endorsements following from the *Soccer Tales Trilogy*.

BOOK REVIEW:

Soccer Tales – Legend of the Shoelace Monster
Posted by Rick Wolff of WFAN Radio
on June 30, 2012

This is a delightful soccer fable that is written with great passion and joy from Lew Freimark. Although aimed for children, it's clearly written in a most unusual and fun manner – and along the way, it introduces the ShoeLace Monster of the soccer pitch.

But this allegorical tale really is the story of Coach Stu and the wonderful time he has had coaching the Vipers through a number of seasons. Author Freimark is able to revisit the history of the game of soccer around the world, and in doing so, he provides a terrific history lesson for all soccer fans, young and old.

Best of all, the content is written in a light and clever approach – there's no sense of heavy-handedness thaf often accompanies kids' books. Bottom line? A fun and different kind of read.

I believe, as caring coaches, parents, and administrators of programs, it is our responsibility to ensure that every child enjoys a positive experience in whatever activity they choose. *"Soccer Tales – Legend of the Shoelace Monster"* is an idyllic journey of joy and teaches life's lessons through children's sports. It says a lot about sports and growing up.

Fred Eng
President and CEO
National Alliance of Youth Sport

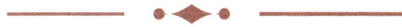

———— •◆• ————

Soccer Tales provide a light-hearted look at soccer and its history. And in the Legend of the Shoelace Monster, young fans are introduced to the passion, the s and the tactics of the beautiful game through an engaging retelling of the exploits of the Vipers soccer team. A good read for new players and young fans-in-the-making.

Phil Schoen, radio host *"The Soccer Show,"* announcer beIN SPORTS, Sirius Radio October, 2017

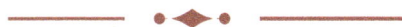

———— •◆• ————

Endorsement for *Soccer Tales III – Baba Yaga's Revenge*, the third installment in the *Soccer Tales Trilogy* from the family of Tony DiCicco, U.S. Women's National Team coach:

"Hi Lew,

I discussed the matter with my family and we decided that yes, you can dedicate the book to our Father. Thank you for honoring him. It is a very fun book, nice job! Thank you for your kind words and thoughts. Best of luck to you!"

Alex DiCicco

———— •◆• ————

A 13 year old's endorsement of *Soccer Tales III*

The Shoo Crew utilizes their knowledge of the game and teamwork to outwit Baba Yaga to save the day. The message reinforces that a soccer player's acumen and teamwork are just as important as their physical or technical ability to play their best.

Nate Bonacci, 13 year old (midfielder, Hillsborough, N.J. soccer club)

———— •◆• ————

The books also have been supported by educators such as Jonathon Vonesh of the Fisher-Climax, Minnesota, girl's basketball team:

"When reading *Soccer Tales I – Legend of the Shoelace Monster* and its sequel, *Soccer Tales II*, I was able to relate to the Vipers and Revolt Teams. My Lady Knights Basketball team of Climax-Fisher, Minnesota had been on a similar journey when they made history. The Lady Knights snapped an 84 game losing streak beating a team in double overtime, with only three players on the court. Victories happen when a team with true HEART, DESIRE, DETERMINATION, PERSE-VERANCE and TENACITY never give up.

———— •◆• ————

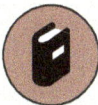

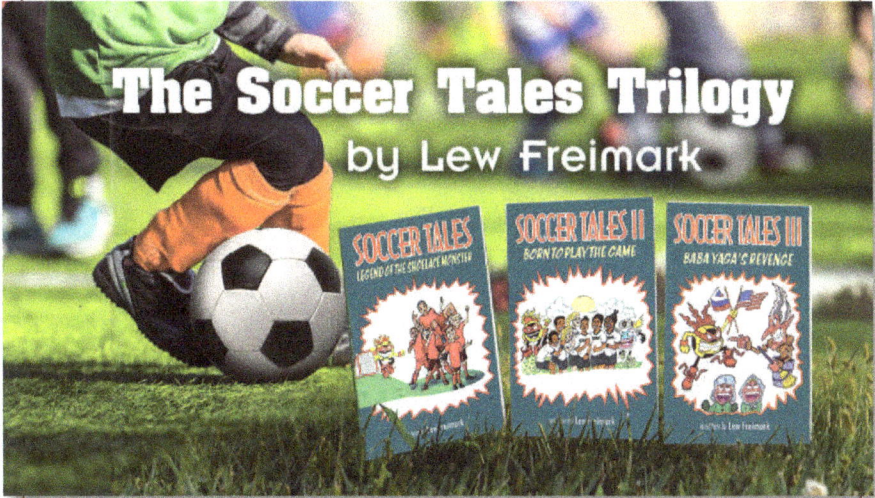